Essays On

Analytical Music Therapy

by

Mary Priestley
LGSM, LGSM (Music Therapy)

Barcelona Publishers

This book is published and distributed by

Barcelona Publishers
1121 N. Rapps Dam Road
Phoenixville PA 19460-1909

© *1994 Barcelona Publishers*

ISBN 0-9624080-2-6

Printed in the United States of America

Cover Illustration
by
Frank McShane

ACKNOWLEDGEMENTS

I extend my grateful thanks to the patients and parents of all the children discussed in this book for giving me their permission to write about our work together. All cases mentioned have had their names and all revealing circumstances altered in order to insure each person's anonymity, and all efforts have been made to preserve the confidentiality of our relationship. It has been an honor for me to work with and learn from each one of them.

My sincere appreciation goes to Dr. Andrew Powell, Dr. J. W. T. Redfearn, Mr. Andrew Samuels, and to Dr. E. G. Wooster for looking through all or parts of the manuscript.

Thanks also to my publisher, long-stop editor and ultimately friend Professor Kenneth Bruscia for standing by postally with weeding trowel, forceps and boiling water to facilitate the final delivery of a disc version of the manuscript. I also thank Ms. Susan Hadley and Ms. Leah Klibanoff, both of Temple University, for their assistance in preparing and proof-reading the final copy of the book.

Thanks are also due to several publishers for permission to use material under copyright. Special appreciation is given to The British Society for Music Therapy and The Association of Professional Music Therapists for allowing me to adapt and reprint articles of mine appearing in the <u>Journal of British Music Therapy</u>. These include:

"Music, Freud and Recidivism" (1977), <u>8</u> (3) 10-14;
"Countertransference in Music Therapy" (1978), <u>9</u> (3) 2-5;
"Music Therapy and Love" (1985), <u>16</u> (3), 2-7; and
"Music and the Listeners: (1988), <u>2</u> (2), 9-13.

These articles appear here as Essays Nine, Eleven, Twenty-Four, and Twenty-Five.

Acknowledgement goes to MMB Music, Inc., in Saint Louis, Missouri for granting permission to reprint Chapters 14-17 (pages 120-152) from <u>Music Therapy in Action</u> (c) 1975 by Mary Priestley. Copyright assigned 1983 to MMB Music Inc.. Additional material (c) 1985 by MMB Music, Inc. Used by Permission. All Rights Reserved. These chapters appear in this book as Essays Three, Four, Five and Six.

Acknowledgement also goes to Gustav Fischer Verlag in Stuttgart Germany for permission to use material based on the following papers of mine which they published:

"Analytische Musiktherapie und Musikalischer Respons," (1980), 1 (1) 21-36;

"Ubertrangung und Genubertragung in der Musiktherapie," (1985), 1 (1/6) 17;

"Musiktherapie in der privaten Praxis," (1985), 6 (4) 287;

"Musiktherapie und Liebe (1986), 7 (1) 1-7.

Thanks are also due to:

---The British Journal of Projective Psychology for their permision to reproduce "Analytical Music Therapy and the Detour Through Fantasy" (1980), 25 (1), 11-14, which appears here as Essay Nineteen;

---The Nursing Times for their kind permission to reproduce "Freud and the Port of Entry" (1976), 72 (49) 1940-1941 which appears here as Essay Seventeen;

---The Guardian newspaper for permission to use some of the material appearing in l/ll/83 Education Guardian; and

---Harper-Collins Publishers of London for permission to quote from A. Storr's Music and the Mind.

Many of these essays originated in the "Herdecke Lectures on Analytical Music Therapy" which I presented in the early 1980's at the Herdecke Community Hospital in Germany. Though originally written in English, these lectures were translated into German by Brigitte Stein and then published in 1983 by The Klett-Cotta Company of Stuttgart Germany under the title Analytische Musiktherapie. I would like to thank Klett-Cotta for their cooperation and support.

Finally, I wish to thank the hotline short-list of those whose advanced or ever-so-slightly-advanced computer know-how helped me to put the book on disc, including: Richard Adeney, Joan Dickson, Charles Hassel, Richard Jasicki, David Michelsen, Peter Michelsen, John Priestley, Joel Wykeham and Dictaphone Ltd..

FOREWORD

These essays were the result of reflective thought and the sifting of feelings about the work I did in two days a week during twenty years at St Bernard's Psychiatric Hospital in London. The hospital has had a tradition of music therapy linked with psychotherapy going back to the year 1955. The work was much helped by my own experience in Kleinian analysis and later Jungian analytical supervision during that time. I was also working in private practice with patients ranging from five-year-old school-phobic children to eminent members of the medical professions. I have had many experiences which I would like to think that through this book I can help younger colleagues to do without.

Some of the essays were based on talks that began the day during four weeks of music therapy training spread over two years at Herdecke Community Hospital in Germany. There I also gave psychodynamic movement and relaxation sessions, instrumental group improvisation work and Intertherapy training.

A background of wartime group singing to keep up morale with my father playing the piano, and playing folkdances for evacuated mothers from London slums in the home my mother ran, professional violin experiences in broadcasting on the Danish Radio, playing for films and in the orchestra pit, and once even busking in the street to clear an unexpected debt, did not prepare me for producing the kind of learned, controlled and scholarly research papers that I proudly see my younger colleagues turning out. Nevertheless I hope that these essays will be of some help to those young music therapists who follow on, polishing the art and keeping alive the eager spirit of exploration and creativity in the service of relieving human distress in our ever-developing profession.

In most of this book I have used the masculine for the therapist and the feminine for the patient to clarify who is doing what. I hope that the readers will not feel upset about this. There are, in fact, at present in this country more female music therapists and psychiatric patients than male, but the numbers are moving towards equalisation in both roles as the financial rewards in the profession improve and the present increasingly unisex approach to home and parental duties introduces our men also to the pull of these conflicting roles.   MP

INTRODUCTION

by

J.W.T. REDFEARN, MA, MD, DPM, DRCPsych.

Over the past years I have been fortunate enough to listen to dozens of Mary Priestley's tape-recordings of musical dialogues with patients and trainees. With the occasional interesting exception, these improvised duets are musically pleasing and sometimes quite beautiful. Most of the patients are musically untrained, yet Mrs. Priestley's assortment of percussive facilities enables them to express emotions directly, simply by using their limbs in a naturally expressive way. The therapist's sensitive response to these expressive noises results in a dialogue and furthermore seems to result in their conversion to music. This is surely analogous to a mother's caring, reflecting response to her infant's babblings and cooings and to the gradual development of a more equal and differentiated relationship between the two as time goes by.

This alchemy whereby noise is transformed towards music, meaninglessness towards meaning, seems to me a most important and striking feature of the work of music therapy. I do not know whether the therapist should aim consciously at this, but there is no doubt that it happens and this happens mainly as a result of harmonious interactions occurring at an unconscious level between therapist and patient.

One tends to take this creative interaction, of which much of the work is being done by the therapist, for granted, until occasionally one hears a recording of a passage or a series of sessions in which such a musical effect is absent. A schizophrenic patient in the early stages of therapy, by subtle change in tonality or rhythm, succeeds in refusing to interact. He makes therapist and listener feel at a loss in a way which no one, however skilled, could imagine to do consciously. Another patient, equally unskilled, using a few simple, repeated notes on the xylophone, manages, again largely unconsciously, to play in such a way as to enable the therapist's piano to hold, playfully nourish, achieve subtle harmonies and changes in rhythm, and together create a beautiful and moving effect. Yet a third, who in his personal relationships has a pattern of intense involvement followed by abandoning the other, has an uncanny tendency to do the very same thing in his therapeutic musical passages. The feeling tone of the product of interaction seems to depend rather little on musical skills, and much more on the emotional qualities of the patient and of his ways of relating. Mrs. Priestley's combination of musical and verbal interaction exposes and clarifies these correlations most effectively.

Why is this? Music is the language of feelings, no doubt because it is rooted biologically in communication through sounds, the communication of the baby's needs to the mother through heartrending wails or infectiously blissful cooings, the need of the frightened member of the group to warn the others, the need to intimidate enemies by roars and harsh sounds, and so on. Music is, perhaps for this reason, quite clearly able both to communicate, and to arouse, almost any depth, quality or intensity of feeling and emotion in people. But, as in the case of the theatre or other art form, the feeling can be dissociated or distanced as necessary.

In other words, we are biologically attuned to react emotionally to sounds of different quality. But the emotional sounds are consonant with other modes of expression. So we are able to pick out the emotionally relevant qualities in our environment through whichever avenue of sensation or perception they reach our awareness. For example, "warmth" can be conveyed: visually (warm colours, warm tones), musically, through the spoken voice, through movements, gestures, expressions of the mouth, expressions in the eyes and their surroundings, touch (e.g. furniture design as well as human contact) and in fact through any avenue, normal and paranormal, into our conscious and unconscious psyche. The term "coenasthesia" is a narrow one to describe this truth, which accounts both for the complexity and the integral nature of our communication and understanding. If I talk of a "noble" wine or speak of Mrs. Priestley's gentle piano holding, playfully caressing, dancing around aggressively, mocking the stodginess of the other's sounds, and so on, I may or may not be right, but I can expect to be understood by anyone but a jackass. The understanding of the patient by the music therapist through the musical dialogue is, has to be made, consonant with the understanding of the patient through whatever biographical or factual data are available. The music therapist, through her musical sensitivity, becomes an emotional sounding-board for the patient, and in the case of Mrs. Priestley at least, can communicate these resonant emotions, reflect them, and help the patient, in words as well as through her music, to understand himself, perhaps even like himself that little bit more, as a result of the musical and verbal exchange.

By the same token, music therapists and therapists of other skills can combine fruitfully in understanding patients, and this has often happened as we have listened to taped sessions and discussed the cases from all angles.

I think it is fair to say that the psychotherapist nowadays has to learn to use the feelings, emotional reactions, and even the instinctual impulses (aggressive, paternal, maternal, loving, and so on) which he finds himself experiencing in relation to the patient, in the further understanding of his patient. In other words, he uses himself and his own emotional reactions to the patient as a kind of emotional or character-divining sounding board. He has to learn to become more sensitive to and aware of, what is going on inside himself in order to gain more knowledge of what is going on in and with his patient. This is far from saying that he must or should enact or express these emotions or burden the patient with them. Often as a therapist one finds oneself thinking or feeling things which seem interesting and perhaps strange or alien to oneself, and one learns to pay attention to these intuitions which often throw light on what is going on in the patient.

transference
counter-transference

The music therapist experiences feelings and emotions, sometimes of a quite specific and detailed sort, through the music she finds herself playing, and should try to make sense of them as part of the data she is accumulating about the patient. Mrs. Priestley brings these (apparently but not actually) subjective experiences to attention in her discussion of countertransference phenomena and their use. Of course, in order to make use of oneself as an emotional sounding board, it could be argued that one ought to be emotionally sound. This requirement would disqualify too many valuable therapists, but at least argues for thorough-going self-knowledge as a necessity if one is to assess these subjective messages.

The expressive-noise-cum-musical dialogue between patient and therapist has mostly to do with the expression of and communication of feelings between them. Feelings can be expressed by both parties which might be too subtle, too embarrassing, or simply too unconscious to be expressed verbally. The immediacy and purity of this feeling interaction is probably unique to music therapy. The time relations of the interaction between patient and therapist are engaged on the same picture. And the therapist in music therapy is always very much there, holding, reflecting, supporting, mollifying, buffeting or otherwise emotionally interacting in a very telling way indeed.

The nonphysical and dissociable nature of the interaction may help in maintaining the best therapeutic working distance and temperature of the interaction. The nonverbal element may provide a point of ingress for the irrational that may be lacking in verbal therapy with some patients. All these considerations may prove important in deciding on the kind of therapy which may be most valuable. But I at least am not ready yet to pontificate about such matters.

The combination of musical sensitivity and psychological interpretative skills possessed by the author of this book must be rare. An artistic family background, a musical, then later a music therapy training, a thorough-going Kleinian analysis, close psychotherapeutic supervision of her work, and many years spent in pioneering her own style of integrating verbal and musical therapy amount to a unique lifetime of preparation for the kind of work she describes in this book. A mere book cannot but whet the appetite for anyone interested in this field, or form a basis for discussion among those wishing to take up this work. I believe this book will perform both these functions well.

Table of Contents

UNIT ONE: FUNDAMENTALS

Door in a High Wall), mythical improvisations, dream work (intracommunication, and dream resolution), and the excercise entitled "Shells, Stones, Sand and Sounds." (From *Music Therapy in Action [1975]*, *pages* 129-136. Reprinted by permission of MMB Music, Inc.).

Defines and gives clinical examples for: reality rehearsals, wholeness, exploring relationships, affirmations and celebrations, subverbal communication, patterns of significance and programmed regression. (From *Music Therapy in Action* [1975], pages 137-145. Reprinted by permission of MMB Music, Inc.).

UNIT TWO: THE THERAPEUTIC RELATIONSHIP

Cites various perspectives on the nature of the therapist-patient relationship, and introduces the "four levels of meeting" in Analytical Music Therapy. (From *Analytische Musiktherapie,* 1983).

Defines and gives clinical examples of the various types of transference and countertransference encountered in Analytical Music Therapy. (From *Musiktherapische Umschau,* 1985, Volume 1, pages 21-36).

Gives more clinical detail on how the analytical music therapist can use empathy and resonance in working with clients. (From *Analytische Musiktherapie,* 1983; and *Journal of British Music Therapy,* 1978, Volume 7 (3), pages 2-5).

UNIT FOUR: THEORETICAL CONCEPTS

Provides clinical and musical examples of basic theoretical constructs of Freud and Klein. (From *Analytische Musiktherapie,* 1983).

Defines and illustrates thirty defenses encountered in Analytical Music Therapy and other psychoanalytically informed therapies. (From *Analytische Musiktherapie,* 1983).

Identifies levels of resistance which are expressed musically and verbally in Analytical Music Therapy. (From *Nursing Times,* 1976, Volume 72, 1940-1941).

UNIT FIVE: THE THERAPEUTIC PROCESS

Examines the various stressors that a patient may experience during therapy, and how the analytical music therapist can deal with them beneficially. (From *Analytische Musiktherapie,* 1983).

UNIT SIX: VARIATIONS

Describes 15 months of Analytical Music Therapy with a married couple in their 60's.

Describes the method for training an analytical music therapist: two trainees take turns with each other in the role of therapist and patient while being observed and supervised by an analytical music therapist. (From *Analytische Musiktherapie*, 1983).

UNIT SEVEN: CADENCE

Describes clinical issues that arise at the end of sessions and/or the treatment itself and possible ways for dealing with them.   (From *Analytische Musiktherapie*, 1983).

A final look at what gives music its special significance and power within the therapeutic process. (From *Analytische Musiktherapie*, 1983).

Essays On

Analytical Music Therapy

Essay One

History and Definition

For some time now I have privately thought that there is no such thing as "Analytical Music Therapy." What I mean by this is that as soon as you think "it is <u>this</u>" or "it is <u>that</u>" you have reified it, concretized it, put it lifeless and inert into a box of words and thus taken it out of the realm of sensitive, spontaneous, empirical creativity which characterizes the therapeutic dyad, and killed it---stone dead. In fact as soon as you can say you have it, you have lost it. It is not <u>this</u> or <u>that</u>, but exists only on the crest of breaking waves of personal musical interaction with a healing bias. To try to describe it is as impossible as trying to give my urban granddaughter the experience of the wonderful blue dragonflies that I saw flitting over a lake in a country garden by taking her to the Natural History Museum and showing her the dried-up specimens of dragonflies under the glass in the display cases.

Nevertheless I must attempt to produce some kind of definition or explanation for analytical music therapy, even though the reader may find a better one after having read through this book---or better still, after having had a few sessions of it.

Analytical Music Therapy (AMT) was developed while I was working as a music therapist with three colleagues in a large psychiatric hospital and while also having my own Kleinian psychoanalysis. AMT was developed to meet the needs of our patients. The first technique - the Splitting Technique - was a direct musical adaptation of the Kleinian theory of splitting which I had experienced through my own analysis. I would have found it impossible to do this just by reading Klein's books. It was my personal experience of the effects of this technique on me during my analysis that inspired me to try and find new music therapy techniques.

Rather than launch out and try this technique on my patients without any experimentation with colleagues, Peter Wright (who was in Jungian analysis) and Marjorie Wardle (who was shortly to start Jungian psychotherapy) and I, formed a triadic "Intertherapy" group. We met in my basement flat weekly for ninety-six sessions trying out different experimental techniques using improvised music, usually on instruments but sometimes also including vocal expression. We usually used a focus in the form of a title with which the mind could direct the emotion.

Although most of the techniques were developed out of our desire to help our patients with their problems, some were the clarification of our own problems following up work that had been done in our analyses. Occasionally something would come from a workshop one of us had attended, thus there are some techniques which nod to Gestalt Therapy and Psychosynthesis. We gave each other feedback on the results of the experimental techniques and I took careful notes in my diary.

Because we thought it better to have a continuation of therapeutic relationships, Peter was Marjorie's therapist, I was Peter's and Marjorie was mine. As Marjorie had not, at that time, had any analysis, I received most of my insights through her sensitive and intuitive use of her piano music backed up by the results of my own analysis.

When, some time later, the publisher Constable commissioned a book on music therapy from me (i.e., Music Therapy in Action), I was at first numb with fright. I put the letter aside for five days in response to one of those paralysing internal objects which seemed to be saying "Of course you can't do it, you've got more than enough to do with having your own analysis, being a single parent to three teenage sons (even if one can be bribed to do the hoovering), doing two days at the psychiatric hospital, having private patients and being in the middle of the Family and Marital Therapy course at the Institute of Group analysis."

On the sixth day I woke up knowing that I wanted to write that book more than anything. The anxiety was not just about writing a book, as I had already had one published about travel, but this was a subject I really believed in and felt strongly about in spite of having had less than five years of the work experience at the time. It was then that I thought of the notes on our Intertherapy sessions and Peter's idea to call our experimental work "Analytical Music Therapy."

My first idea was that this collection of techniques and experiences called Analytical Music Therapy was something that one learnt, then had, and maybe eventually received a Diploma for, which one could put in a frame alongside the others hanging on one's music room wall. However, when the book came out and the Intertherapy students came along in pairs, I realised that this was an orientation training to a certain way of working using one's whole life experience, together with one's own analysis or analytical psychotherapy as a skeleton on which to hang ideas about what developed between the therapist, patient and the music. I was impressed and delighted at the individuality of each student's response to the training and their subsequent use of it in their university and other teaching posts abroad.

After a time I heard from ex-Intertherapy students that certain German analysts did not like the title and so I nervously changed it to Exploratory Music Therapy to please these faceless critics. I would happily have called it "Humpty Dumpty" if I was referred more private patients as its use seemed to be helping our hospital patients. However, when my analysis was over, my Jungian supervisor, Dr. J. W. T. Redfearn said that, since this title was already in a book he did not see why it should not remain as it was. And so it did.

Having been a psychiatric patient myself at the age of twenty-two (1947), when treatments were rather cruder and extremely frightening, I had a tremendously anxious respect for the opinions of doctors, and due to early relegation of home-parenting to nurses, I also had an irrational but lingering horror of anything female that went by that title.

So Analytical Music Therapy is the name that has prevailed for the analytically-informed symbolic use of improvised music by the music therapist and client. It is used as a creative tool with which to explore the client's inner life so as to provide the way forward for growth and greater self-knowledge. The analytical music therapist, a qualified musician and music therapist to start with, (though there have also been a few German doctors and psychiatrists with musical qualifications), will have been trained in the Intertherapy orientation course, having previously or subsequently had personal experience of analysis or analytical psychotherapy. A few analytical music therapists have done a more body-based, post-post-postgraduate personal training based on the work of a former Freudian.

Peter and Marjorie were, and are at the time of writing, fine pianists involved also in accompaniment and therefore highly trained in playing and listening.   As a violinist, my experience of chamber music also helped me in this way; and though I developed a way of improvising on the piano which one of my German colleagues amazed me by describing as brilliant, I never actually went higher than Grade Four at the Royal College of Music in this second study.   I am admitting this as I thought it might help another would-be analytical music therapist whose piano performance and sight reading may be less than wonderful.

Hearing about music therapy for the first time people usually leap to the quotation about music soothing the savage breast, however, AMT does not always aim at instantly producing good experiences, as it is often necessary to work through the emotionally painful blockages before going forward with one's development.   This may then allow such good experiences to occur in the way that best suits the client and allows her to feel strengthened and validated by them.   Obviously one must to a certain extent be guided by the patient and her motivation, her residue of hope and courage and her will to progress.

An interesting analogy on the physical level is the experience of the very testing pain in a Qigong class when the Chi is making its way through a blocked meridian.   Our teacher, when asked what one could do about it, just smiled the amazing real-teeth Chinese smile and said, "Put up with it.   It vanishes quite suddenly." And it did.

Within the AMT session such rewarding good experiences could be a sudden strongly positive and affirmative (often early preverbal) memory that a patient has, knowing that at that particular remembered moment she was deeply and truly beloved, whatever may have happened in the development of that primal relationship later.   It could also be the joy of being able to share nonverbally with the therapist a life-enhancing inner or outer happening, the experience of harmonious and beautiful rhythmic interaction, or the reassurance of being able to survive a wildy chaotic or dissonant musical interaction and end in peace and friendship.   Occasionally and awesomely, it can be the dawning realisation of the root cause of a continuing truth-distorting "beta statement" (Bion, 1977)---or what I call a "not yet consciously considered action or motivation resulting from an early trauma that has continued to resonate terrifyingly to quite seemingly in-ocuous events in the present, triggering off violent and embarrassing emotional storms" (p. 72). This can be followed by the realisation of how infinitely understandable and forgivable that event was when seen from the present adult level. Another good experience can be the pleasure of moving to one's own recorded improvised duet music in a session, and letting the kinaesthetic awareness bring further insights. Sometimes it is just sitting together in chosen silence feeling the harmonious non-necessity of words until the time feels right to speak.

Outside the session these experiences could lead to the search for better and more satisfying relationships and experiences, the determination and hard work entailed in eliminating at least the worst of the residual destructive and crippling trauma resonances along with their accompanying body tensions still operating in the present, and the courage to be more self-assertive and self-expressive without the need to be destructive or insensitive to the feelings of others. Of course, this is a tall order while also being a quite useful direction for the rest of one's life.

Along with these good experiences, however, there can be difficult interludes, often caused by having to face the release of the previously frozen emotional pain. But having someone on your side helps to make these experiences assimilable, even more so if the person is properly trained him/herself and is therefore not asked to try and help for 168 hours a week without an understanding of how to do this.

Music in this therapy is used in its four aspects: vocal, instrumental, movement with the body-as-instrument, and selective silence, all of which bring an awareness of one's own inner music as well as music of wider spheres.

Now it is necessary to look at what Analytical Music Therapy is not. First, it is not merely a type of music lesson. The results of successful music therapy should be looked for in the quality of the patient's life and being, and not in the improvement in the quality of her musical improvisation or performance, unless this is her considered life aim. Indeed her music may be the one factor that shows little or no change at all after as much as five years of quite successful therapeutic work. It can be a kind of pedal point that gives the security that allows for change and growth in many other areas. This is not always the case, for some clients are musically creative too.

Second, AMT is not psychoanalysis, although there are some

similarities. For example the analysand lies on the couch, unable to view her analyst directly, and obeys the fundamental rule: to free-associate and keep nothing back that comes to mind. The Analytical Music Therapist's patient (or client if she is not having psychiatric treatment) opens herself to a deeper or shallower extent in their musical duet, and is invited to communicate by sharing her feelings, inner experiences and thoughts with the therapist after they have finished playing, however weird, shocking or shameful these may seem. But, unlike in analysis, there is a lively, emotional reciprocity between therapist and client through the musical duet improvisation, and this carries over to a certain extent into their exchange in words.

Third, AMT is not a magic therapy or instantaneous healing which will give either the therapist or patient the power to transcend all problems and difficulties without focussed work. It is a form of treatment with its own limitations and contraindications like any other. But unlike a mechanical form of treatment it depends very much for its success on the knowledge, skill, warmth, power and depth of the personality of the therapist, the willingness of the client to work on herself, the rapport between them and the reasonable support of her home environment.

Lastly, analytical music therapy is not the experimental use of the techniques outlined in <u>Music Therapy in Action</u> (Priestley, 1975) by therapists who have not themselves explored their own inner lives musically with another analytical music therapist, as happens in the Intertherapy training. To submit others to these techniques without having experienced anything of their power on oneself is irresponsible dabbling and could be dangerous. The world of dreams and imagination in which we operate is also the strange world of psychosis; it is not so difficult to enter but the therapist must also know the way out--- and back to the awareness of the life of the everyday world. This is important both for himself, and his private patients, who will also have to leave the shelter of the treatment room and make their way home in an alert frame of mind while crossing streets of a busy city.

Personally I find there is no other therapy so helpful with the decoding of the personal message and usefulness of dreams, and still seek out my original Intertherapy partner to work on my own dreams now and then. If I find myself at all disenchanted with the work of

AMT, I have only to go back for a few personal sessions to be full of enthusiasm and excitement about it again.

In Analytical Music Therapy the guided expression of the music seems, in many cases, to reduce the patient's resistance to denied or split-off emotion as it can lower the threshold of consciousness. It allows this emotion to be experienced symbolically in sound or movement and therefore a little less painfully. Often this expression brings with it vivid memories and inner images. Some people have a deep fear at the thought of releasing repressed material from the unconscious. But they do not understand that unconscious hidden impulses can have much stronger and more unpleasant effects on a person's life and the lives of those around her when they are still in the unconscious. Here they can be the cause of unpleasant symptoms, irrational fears, inexplicable moods and sometimes serious crimes. Indeed, several murderers, who I have met in the course of my work, seemed to be the kind of meek person who would not hurt a fly until one day the pent up rage erupted, often through being goaded by a house-sharing relative.

An impulse thus released during therapy can either be accepted or partly accepted, or it can be sublimated and used in a constructive, creative and harmless way, or it can be consciously condemned. Either way it frees a good deal of energy which was formerly used in keeping it unconscious. The process working against the release of such impulses Freud termed the "resistance."

This might be the place briefly to look at the concept of the resistance as Freud explained it. Imagine attending a lecture and a member of the audience becoming obstreperous and causing a disturbance. Then imagine that two other members put him outside, put chairs in front of the door and sit on them. The audience here represents the conscious mind, the place outside the unconscious mind; the unruly member is the impulse; and the two members seated by the door constitute the resistance. Now if another member of the audience approaches the door, persuades the recalcitrant member to go quietly back to his seat, and succeeds in asking the two seated members to move aside, then he is playing the part of the therapist.

Another important use of analytical music therapy is that through the musical expression aggressive and auto-aggressive tendencies can be externalised in sound expression without the therapist succumbing to the assault.   This relieves the patient of the guilt of having to create verbal channels of hate and destructiveness which might be better left unverbalised.   This can, in time, lead to the positive use of aggression as assertiveness in the acquisition of valuable life aims, although the patient will often initially need to be guided through a phase of an uneasy use of this externalised aggression.

As an example of this externalisation of auto-aggression I cite the case of a 30 year old married school teacher with a form of manic-depressive illness. I treated her in hospital as an adjunct to her chemotherapy and as an out-patient afterwards. She used to get attacks of a painful unreal feeling (depersonalisation) and then slash her wrists to convince herself that she was really there. She told me that she felt that there was a barrier between her and other people, especially her husband. She had described this as a pane of thick glass and in fact she had smashed several panes of glass both in her home and in the street at around that time.   In our improvisation we took the title "Breaking down the Barrier." All the violence which she had formerly turned against herself was vented on the instruments. She pounded so hard on the xylophone that all the note bars bounced off and she then threw them violently all over the music room. She clashed on the cymbal in a frenzy and then took it down on the floor and with amazing strength twisted it into the shape of a sombrero hat. I may say that this was on a dark winter night when our Portakabin was a long way from any kind of help should it be needed.

When all this was done, my double-forte, containing piano music stopped and we sat silent for some time amid the wreckage of scattered xylophone bars and battered instruments. Only minutes later, when she began to pick up the wreckage, did I follow her lead. (I was determined that she should not project her controlling Super-ego on to me, but should be in control of herself).   Together we silently re-created order in the room. In spite of everything we still had a good working alliance. She offered to replace the cymbal. I thanked her and she brought a new one to the next session.

This attack was an outburst of infantile anger, the bending of the cymbal being possibly a symbolic attack on the mother's breast. My quiet response was a model aimed at teaching the patient that she could contain such feelings and cope with them without disasters happening. This marked the turning point of her aggression changing into assertion in goal-seeking. She gradually became able to be more assertive in life. She learnt to drive a car and bought one for herself. She took a huge class of children for drama at school and successfully produced an entertainment. After some marital therapy with a social worker and myself, the patient and her husband decided to separate. With some colleagues she took a party of deprived children on an adventure holiday pot-holing in caves, riding, cliff-climbing, and hiking, and she organised a satisfactory social life.

Our music was not a magic spell creating all this, but we did meet musically at the moment when she tested out whether it was safe to unleash her unused energy, formerly turned against herself, on to the outside world. Our experience marked the turning point of its re-direction. Now, some seventeen years later, I still get the annual Christmas card with news of her successful work with mentally handi-capped children overseas.

In the introduction to Music Therapy in Action (Priestley, 1975), Dr. E. G. Wooster described how in AMT, the healthy parts of the patient can come to work with such "mad" parts as dissociated impulses or perceptions, groundless fears, bodily symptoms, or rigid, defensive structures. He wrote that in hospitals, patients are often considered as wholly mad, and so their sane and healthy parts do not ordinarily get a chance to help their "mad" parts. Frequently when they meet these "mad" parts they find that they, too, have their reason and can be understood and perhaps even alleviated.

For example, a mechanical engineer of 32 (see chapter 21 of Music Therapy in Action) was referred to me by his psychiatrist. The patient had had inexplicable back pains for which he had been treated in vain with chemotherapy for two years. Throughout this time he had been off work. With the aid of our music he got in touch with the message of the pains. These were interpreted as the psychosomatic expression of his anger about the symbolic stabs in the back by the cruel breasts of the mother who had abandoned the little family when he was four. It took two more years of working through his anger, bitterness and fears before he was ready to work outside again. But during his music therapy treatment he worked full time in the Industrial

Unit. His illness had come on when his own son reached the age of four and unconsciously he felt that if he did not stay at home, he, in identification with his son, would be abandoned, this time by his wife, his son's mother.

It might be helpful here to give some idea of the typical AMT session and how the work is arranged. The therapist usually, but not inevitably, starts the session by listening to the client, what she has been feeling and thinking about and doing, and how she has been getting on. With a few patients this can degenerate into a defensive chatter designed to lead the attention away from any true feelings and serious problems. This can be spoken about, but with such patients it is often better to begin with an untitled duet improvisation between client and therapist, who play five to ten minutes to see what the music brings up. However, normally the therapist will be in touch with the music that is behind the words.

For example, an office worker suffering from manic-depressive illness came to her session talking about difficulties with the office manager. Behind these words and the quite realistic troubles was the music of a child's distress, a child who felt wronged. Our musical improvisation brought out memories of difficulties with the "managers" at home in her early life.

During the first session the therapist will take the client's history in quite a comprehensive way so that he has all the facts written down for later reference and for use in case studies or supervision. Otherwise he will not take notes in a patient's session but wait until afterwards. After some talk, and possibly some silence, when there seems to be something that they can explore together, they go to the instruments. The client will sit by a battery of instruments such as a chromatic xylophone, a 16" tom-tom, a 12" cymbal on a stand, a gong, melodica, bells (on my home-made bell tree), tambourine and so on. Sometimes the therapist will ask the client what she wants to play about but often the therapist will pick a subject, or two roles, from the client's material which the client herself would not only not choose, but would most probably studiously avoid because it might lead to a blocked area.

The therapist usually plays the piano as she has more control of the situation with the harmony and volume of this instrument.

Naturally the client's voice can be considered as an extra instrument if she is not too inhibited to use it, and again she can move expressively to the recording of her own improvised music using the body as an instrument if that feels possible and natural. I suspect that the clients of the future will enter more easily into these ways of self-expression when the many cultures in this one-time island begin to blend more harmoniously and more frequently.

The therapist's function in this duet is twofold. He will, with his musical expression, contain the emotion of the client, matching her honest moods. He must also be alert to that inner voice from the client's unconscious: the countertransference (see essays 8 and 9); and sometimes reproduce musically these feelings from the client's unconscious. The countertransference (used here not in the sense of the therapist's distorting transference on to the patient but also of his reactions to the patient's unconscious or preconscious feelings) is a useful tool for exploring the client's hidden emotion and it is made more reliable by the therapist previously having gone through the process of analysis and analytical music therapy in the client position and exploring his inner life musically so that he does not confuse his own feelings with his reactions to those of his client. Initially this sensitivity may develop slowly and it may take time for the therapist to have the confidence to trust in the validity of these messages and use them fruitfully in his therapy. Most music therapists, or musically-trained doctors and psychiatrists who have had Intertherapy training, have found that the period of analytical psychotherapy before or after the Intertherapy was extremely helpful, too, especially in dealing with the verbal side of the therapy.

After they have finished playing, the client may talk about her inner and outer experiences, and the therapist may say what he thought about the music (sometimes as a model for how freely one can talk about these personal experiences) and then the tape is played back. Astonishingly enough, although seldom musically trained, patients can almost always recognise the exact spot, in this fragmented melange of tones and rhythms, where a certain inner image or feeling occurred. Often, too, in the playback they are aware of the therapist's music for the first time and this can be very reassuring. This can also be linked to the experience of the small child feeling confident held in his mother's arms but not yet aware of being held.

I am sometimes asked whether clients object to me recording their music. In fact I do not ask them whether they object or not but only explain that it is useful for us to hear our music and necessary for me to keep records. I do not record their voices and I explain this. No one has ever complained about this and when I have asked their permission to play their music to a case conference or for a broadcast, only one has ever complained in 25 years. Working in the psychiatric hospital I only once, when intending to record a group session, had a patient in the paranoid schizophrenic state who imagined that the machine was going to suck the life out of her. In that case we did not record, out of respect for her feelings rather than agreement with her delusion.

The therapist relates to the patient in an inner way through intuition and an outer way through the ears and eyes. The inner way is called countertransference. As an example of the action of counter-transference: I had referred to me, by a consultant psychotherapist, a man in his early thirties who worked with a commercial concern. He was mildy schizophrenic and had been given to falling into catatonic states. He wanted us to play a musical conversation between himself and a client at work and then himself and a colleague. We improvised and, through the countertransference, I found myself overtaken by such a strange, dreamy feeling that I seemed to be playing in a trance. I said to him afterwards that I felt that I was playing the music of a part of him that was concerned neither with colleagues nor with clients. He then admitted that he had a secret dream that he nourished at work. It was of being able to burst marvellously into song, anywhere and everywhere. We talked about the glorious feeling of the power to ravish with delight and the unsteadying omnipotence, and decided that he should vocalise in one of our improvisations each week in future. That countertransference feeling did not the recur.

So much for the execution of the AMT technique. Now for details of its practice. In 1979 there were forty trained analytical music therapists spread over Britain, Germany, Denmark., Austria, Canada and the U.S.A. In 1978 the German analytical music therapists, sponsored by their Ministry of Science and Research, ran a two year Mentorkursus Musiktherapie concentrating on the methods of Nordoff-

Robbins and analytical music therapy. Students experienced the latter method in the patient role at first and later formed Intertherapy pairs supervised by tutors trained in AMT. The course took place at the well-known Herdecke Community Hospital with periods of practical work in hospitals in Britain, Holland and Germany. The resident tutors were Professors Johannes Eschen, Ole Teichmann-Mackenroth and Colleen Purdom, all of whom graduated in the music therapy course at the Guildhall School of Music in London and took the Intertherapy analytical music therapy training with me afterwards.

This training has been given privately in London, the trainees coming in pairs, experiencing AMT in the client position first, and later coming together and taking turns to be therapist and client to each other under my personal supervision. A programme of reading and discussion complimented the practical work.

No rigorous control-group tests have been carried out with AMT patients, and, in fact, I think it would be difficult to do this, because of the personal element on one side and the fact that most of the hospitalised patients who formed the bulk of our intake were having additional therapies such as chemotherapy, art therapy, occupational therapy, drama therapy, social skills, religious counselling or intense experiences with the foot care assistants. Therapists practising new techniques tend to be sent patients who have been found untreatable by other means; Freud had the same complaint during his early days, and wrote about it in one of his last papers.

There are certain guidelines about patient suitability for analytical music therapy. Patients experiencing extreme deafness might be suitable but I personally have had no experience with them. Patients who have an IQ below 80 have been treated with some success by colleagues but I think that here also specialist knowledge and experience would be demanded of the therapist. However, the regular analytical music therapist can practise a simpler, more descriptive style of therapy with such patients and, indeed, their IQ has often been kept artificially low by their emotional blocks to thinking. Overtly psychotic patients who are experiencing a world of dreams, called hallucinated and deluded, are already living symbolically which precludes the conscious understanding of symbols as such. If a manic-depressive or schizophrenic patient becomes overtly psychotic during treatment, the therapist can resort to a simpler technique until the patient is able to distinguish between the dream world of symbols and the world of everyday life. There is no danger in using Analytical Music Therapy with such patients; it is merely unprofitable in its more sophisticated state during the period of their psychotic functioning. The totally split kind of psychopathic patient must be handled very cautiously, my experience with this rarer type of patient in prison is very limited as I was only a locum therapist. I am sure there is room for more careful work to be done here on a longterm basis.

There have been some encouraging results. A middle-aged lady with a history of seven years of agoraphobia was free of the symptom after four months of AMT, together with help from the Psychology Department. A young mother, estranged from her second daughter, worked on these feelings with music. Through this work she managed to withdraw from the child the displacement of hostile feelings which belonged to the patient's sister with similar hair colouring, whom the patient had found in bed with her (the patient's) husband. A young wife recovered from long-standing frigidity after 16 sessions. A wife and mother recovered from a 16 year old phobia, which had stopped her from working even voluntarily, in 32 sessions. A hemiplegic man who had not been employed for 15 years started a new career after 88 sessions. The conversion hysteric, who I described earlier, who had had psychiatric treatment without success for two years (when he was at home off work) went back to full time employment after 96 session during which time he worked at the Industrial Training Unit. These are just a few examples.

Of course, there have been some failures too, earlier on some patients who developed a negative transference opted out of therapy before this could be worked through. Even in successful cases, some patients can go through very difficult phases, suffering from deeply painful emotions and sometimes needing extra support from the therapist or the environment. However, where improvement does occur, for whatever reason, it is in the direction of freer self-expression and a feeling of balance in its use; increased self-respect; a more focussed sense of purpose in their lives; diminution or greater toleration of psychosomatic symptoms; quicker recovery from emotional disturbances; increase in adventurousness (many patients end up getting better jobs); more satisfying relationships and some increase in energy for life.

I will conclude with two paragraphs from the introduction to Music Therapy in Action (Priestley, 1975) by my analyst, the Consultant Psychotherapist and Group Analyst, Dr. E. G. Wooster, who did so much to pilot us pioneer analytical music therapists through our initial difficulties.

Carrying out the techniques of analytical music therapy is not as easy as it may sound. Many psychotic reactions are based on a denial of that which is painful in the outer or inner world. A great many neurotics, too, would rather keep their phobic, obsessional or psychosomatic mechanisms - to name but a few - rather than trade them in for the deep anxieties and guilts which lie hidden beneath them.

The naive therapeutic enthusiast, who succeeds in prising open a patient's defences in order to let their repressed anger or sexuality have an airing by musical, verbal or any other means, is likely to be given a bloody nose - metaphorically or actually - resulting in the patient's exacerbated need to say 'I told you so' as he reinforces his defences even more strongly. Such a patient feels (often unconsciously) that since, in the past, his attempts to express himself were punished or went unrewarded, he is going to need to experience his attempts in the here-and-now very differently in order to allow himself to question his previous assumptions about the result of self-expression. This would be true in any therapeutic situation, including that of music therapy (p. 13).

Essay Two

Getting Started
With a Patient

The main aim in getting started with a patient is to make a relationship. It will most probably be a relationship of a kind that the patient has never experienced before---one which, on the one hand, gives her opportunities to be herself and discover herself in a quite new way; and on the other hand, demands a very great deal of her in that she will be relating to the therapist on different levels.

To take the first point, the patient will experience a quality of listening that she has surely not had before or she would most likely not be in therapy. The therapist will be taking in not only the facts but also the feelings about these facts---feelings which the patient may not yet realise that she has. This will be a nonretaliatory, nonpunitive and noncompetitive relationship. Even though angry and violent wishes may be thrown at the therapist, he will not retaliate but will aim at unearthing the hurt and sad feelings that lie behind them. Dr. Franz Alexander called this a "corrective emotional experience" in that it supplied that understanding and tolerance of the patient's emotional life which was missing in her early life.

To come to the second point: the patient will be required to relate to the therapist on three different levels. First there is the rational adult-to-adult level which forms the "working alliance." On this level the patient brings herself to the session regularly, if she is a private patient she makes herself responsible for payment and she is responsible for relieving her more violent feelings at a verbal or musical level rather than acting them out in wild actions in, or outside, therapy.

Next there is the subverbal musical level where the emotions of the therapist and patient mingle freely together in music and there is a certain circumscribed level of acting out of strong feelings on the instruments. Lastly there is the transference relationship in which the patient re-plays child-to-parent feelings with the therapist and thereby is able to re-enact, interpret and subsequently alter the earlier relationships. The therapist who is working with the transference will clarify what is happening in the present and relate it to what happened in the

past.   After some working on the feelings when they arise, and
understanding the behaviour they produce, they no longer return
unbidden and destructively, as they do when the unconscious tries to
distort present and future relationships. This can, understandably be
a long process entailing hard work on both sides.

The patient's first communication to the therapist is very
important. He must be aware that there is something that the patient
wishes to share, some direction that she wants to follow but at the
same time there will be a counter-direction, a resistance to this
direction. Jung said that every patient has a secret and that until it is
told she cannot regain her health. However, many patients have strong
motives for not wanting to recover. Their illness gives them secondary
gains such as the solicitude and attention of their nearest relatives; and,
the challenges and stresses of a normal, healthy life are no compensa-
tion for the lack of this anxious concern. The balance of these warring
valences will be weighed and worked on by the therapist as he gets the
feeling of the patient's personality.

The physical arrangement of the therapy room is also quite
important.   There are certain advantages in having the two chairs
facing one another about two or three meters apart. In this way the
therapist has access not only to the spoken words of his patient but also
her unconscious body messages which often keep the communication
going when the patient's words have dried up, or not yet begun to
flow. These can be silently read and noted, or they can be interpreted
as a separate but complimentary language. For example, a forty-year
old manic depressive woman used to fall silent and cover the top of her
head with her arms. She looked like a child warding off a blow to the
head. I told her this and gradually her parents' punitive attitude to her
childish incontinence came to light together with her anger, indignation
and shame.

When the therapist and patient move over to the instruments,
too, there must be the possibility of eye contact, as very important
revelations are often made after the patient has been playing. For this
reason it is useful for the therapist to sit on a swivelling chair rather
than on a piano stool.   Special attention should be paid to body
messages via the instruments after the improvisation has been played
i.e. the holding of the xylophone beaters during speech. This can be

particularly revealing. For example, a periodically depressed patient of 41 felt very threatened by getting close to people emotionally. She played some music depicting loving feelings but afterwards sat holding the two beaters in one hand but with a finger between them. From this I got a clue that she was afraid of getting too close to me because of her disastrous relationships with her parents, both of whom committed suicide. She was offering me some symbolic magical protection because she feared unconsciously that her love could kill.

An obsessional neurotic man of 36, who was single, was expressing each emotion in turn on the xylophone with a beater in each hand. When he came to Love, he transferred the two beaters to his right hand. He felt ready for a close relationship.

An impotent man of 47 sat with his legs apart and the two beaters held between them like an erect phallus. When he got excited while talking he made some violent masturbatory movements up and down the sticks. This gave the clue that a masturbatory phantasy might be blocking the establishment of a normal relationship with his wife.

It is essential to take notes on sessions not only for one's own use for the writing up or presenting of an eventual case study, but also, in these quarrelsome days, for proof of what transpired in a certain session when even what instruments were being used is asked for by the investigators of malpractice. However, I only advise writing notes during the session at the time of the first session when one must have a record of all kinds of facts and phone numbers that one will need to refer to later. Otherwise it is better to take notes after the session. The one exception to this is with dreams. Dreams, with their different characters and symbolic shapes and colours of objects, can be particularly difficult to remember for therapists who do not have a keen visual memory and the ability to recreate the scene described in their minds over and over again at will. In fact I have found patients rather proud to have their dreams recorded in this way, it somehow makes them more substantial and worthy of serious attention. And, as Jung mentioned, when dreams get more serious attention the dreamer is awarded better dreams.

For the first session I have found it useful to have a questionnaire which can be used by the therapist as a skeleton on which to base the gathering of information. In the first meeting I open myself in a particular intuitive way to patients, often seeing inner pictures which are symbolically relevant to their situation. This way of functioning makes it difficult for me to think in a logical rational way what should come next and what I might have missed out that was vital for the first session. Thus, the questionnaire helps me a great deal.

It took me many years to create the questionnaire but I believe that it is now a very useful aid to the first session; so much so that a younger colleague of mine, to whom I gave it, went through it with one mature male patient who said that now he could see just what was wrong with his life and did not feel the need to do more work on it musically. Naturally one does not bark out the questions like a newly empowered official but first of all the patient will be encouraged to speak freely about herself and her difficulties. Later the areas which are still in the dark can be examined with questions. Each question should be given in as open-ended a form as possible to give the patient the opportunity to continue her train of thought. It is important that she be allowed to answer in the way that she chooses even if the therapist has to come back and pick up lost information afterwards to complete the picture of the background. However, there is a conflict here between letting her tell her story undisturbed (even if you do not quite understand one or another point) and stopping to clarify a point which seems vital to the true understanding of the situation even if it does interrupt the flow.

For example, one of the questions asked is about the patient's siblings. This question might lead to a long story about one of the older siblings who was preferentially treated, at the end of this the therapist would have to ask about the three younger siblings who were not even going to be mentioned. But the first story was necessary. Curiously enough, I have found that no patients vouchsafe their siblings' names at first. Perhaps there is always felt to be too much sharing and competition for attention with them already. Therefore if the therapist can get the relative ages of the siblings that is probably enough for the first session. Later their names can be taken down and this can be very useful in refreshing one's memory before a session.

There is a question about groups, which is to cover social relationships and also membership of clubs, religious organisations and so on. Most of my patients have been loners, however, some have belonged to certain strict religious bodies, and in these cases, some knowledge of rules and taboos was vitally important to our work. For example, one Catholic patient who had never resolved her feelings about her parents' deaths, was very upset and insecure at the time of the two Popes' deaths. Her feeling of abandonment was so great that she retaliated by stopping the therapy. Since her mother had been very depressed, in a sense she had never had anything but abandonment.

The questions about the family will not only tell you something about the social class and background of the patient but will bring out the feeling tones of various relationships and the family patterns and myths, which in turn will alert you as to what to expect in the transference. For example, a patient who was seduced by an older relative not only was on the look-out for seduction by me but used to reverse the roles. In the role of the relative she would try and seduce me out of the therapist-patient relationship with frequent delightfully seductive gifts and familiar talk on the way out of the session.

Another patient of 19, who had conversion hysteria, was a twin in a family of eight siblings. She talked at a tremendous rate as if trying not to leave the slightest gap for any other person to enter her session. After this was interpreted many times, some of the pressure in her speech was reduced, but her xylophone playing remained quite frenetic and prestissimo during our several years of work together.

Four common taboo areas---money, sex, death and psychic or spiritual experiences---are touched on in the questionnaire. With an institutionalised patient there will be less need to discuss money but sometimes, at some point, it can be quite useful to let the patient know what the treatment would cost if she was having it privately.

Sex is a subject which is delicate at any age. The therapist will endeavour to create a climate where feelings about this aspect of the relationship can be explored symbolically in music or openly in words as freely as with any other subject. Not knowing whether it is relevant or acceptable to the therapist, many patients tend to withold information on this subject unless a definite lead is given by the therapist. Whether the first session is the right time to give that lead is a question each therapist must decide for himself. But certainly he should be asking himself what is being done with this patient's sex drive, whether it is contributing to a loving relationship, being sublimated into creative channels, being repressed and returning as symptoms, seducing the patient into a secret life of phantasy and guilt, or being used sadistically as a vehicle of rage, fear and revenge.

Death, and especially mourning, is dealt with better in some countries than in others. In modern Western society it is an event which can create emotion that others find hard to deal with and so the bereaved person can easily become isolated, encapsulated and scotomised, causing a dangerous dissociated area of grief, anger and often unjustifiable guilt.

Recent research by the Alister Hardy Research Centre for Spiritual experiences revealed that a great many people have had strange experiences of this kind which they feared to speak about as no one else did, and they did not like to be thought peculiar. Whether one calls them psychic, spiritual or glimpses into the unconscious is not so important as being able to share this side of the patient's experience which otherwise might make her feel very isolated. In a hospital meeting I actually heard a psychiatrist say that the patient under discussion must be psychotic because she believed in God (which, of course, puts the Pope and Archbishop of Canterbury in quite an unsettling situation)!

The therapist will open these areas sensitively to help the patient to realise that this therapeutic relationship is unlike others that she may have had and that it is possible within this relationship to think and talk about things that could not be expressed elsewhere as they might there cause derision, shock, disgust or punitive responses. Needless to say, if this initial exploration is done without sensitivity this could do more harm than good. If the therapist has not had his own taboo areas sufficiently lighted up and finds that he cannot open up such topics at all, then he or she may need to have further group or individual analytical psychotherapy or music therapy to help him to feel more at ease in the therapist role.

Questions about drugs, alcohol and sleeping are especially relevant in the private setting where the therapist could risk receiving the patient in an inebriated state or in an amphetamine psychosis. Changes in the sleep pattern often precede serious emotional illness and should be gone into, together with a discussion on evening lifestyle, before sending the patient off to the general practioner for sleeping pills. Incidentally some nursing homes for elderly people are finding that aroma therapy and a little massage at night is eliminating the need for the old automatic sleeping pill routine.

If the patient or her psychiatrist lets the therapist know what medication she is taking, he can acquaint himself with the side effects. Doctors often do not tell the patients about these because they are afraid that their patients will stop taking the drugs or start imagining side effects that they might not have noticed. But I have found that more patients have been made anxious because they thought that the various side effects of dry mouth, blurred vision giving a disinclination to read, shaky hands and so on were an indication of some other sinister physical disease which they sometimes did not even dare ask about. When they learned that these were side effects they were able to arrange their lives accordingly for example listening to more "Talking Books" instead of reading as much as before, sucking peppermints instead of drinking gallons of water and such things.

Questions about the patient's musical history can be a fruitful line of enquiry. Finding out which parent played the instrument that they learnt can lead to the discovery of helpful identifications on the one hand, or pressurising living-out of the parent's unfulfilled ambitions on the other hand. Which sibling played the same instrument can open up talk about rivalry. However, often musically-proficient amateurs do not make easy clients for analytical music therapy. They do not always take to improvising their feelings freely in sound painting, as they prefer to show off their proficiency by playing the feelings of Mozart or Haydn, especially in a group.

The patient's self-evaluation provides important clues for her self-image. Sometimes it is a very harsh part of the self judging a masochistic part. For example, a 36 year old man with mood swings described himself as "moody, serious and a pain in the arse." The last phrase had probably been used or indicated by the grandmother who brought him up. A 41-year old American musician, who had had six years of Jungian analysis, had a much more generous view of herself: "emotional, highly strung, intense, having humour and gaiety, mood swing, sometimes depressed otherwise capable and warm". The idealised and grandiose self-image, usually polarised with acute feelings of inferiority, is often revealed by this question.

When you have listened to the patient's view of herself and asked your questions, it is wise to ask whether there is anything else relevant that she thinks you ought to know. It can be surprising what new material this can produce. For example, a well-educated hysterical woman of 54 told the therapist that she was unable to pass exams. This had led to a lifetime of doing menial office jobs which had contributed to the fact that she had been unable to find friends of her own class and, being rather snobbish, this had made her into a very solitary person.

Right from the start, even though the therapist may need to ask some questions, the relationship between the therapist and the patient should, basically, be that of the "container" to the "contained." If she is faced with a therapist who can contain all her emotion without retaliation, she will have a model that she may later on be able to take into herself, enabling her to contain her own and probably her children's or employees' emotion when necessary. This may be the container that she has never had before and which may be crucial for her growth towards wholeness.

And now we come to music. The deep subverbal layer of the musical exchange needs to be carefully prepared. The language of free, atonal or modal improvisation is almost always totally strange to the patient. It cannot profitably be explained. It is not a cerebral exercise but a response to feelings which may have been hidden for decades. The patient must somehow instantly discover and use this technique as a channel of communication for these feelings. Once she has done this and felt the relief of this expression and the satisfaction in the creativity, this third kind of relationship will become operative.

The first improvisation is very important. Is the patient going to find this a helpful, releasing containing experience for her emotions, or will it be an embarrassing, difficult or even impossible task? The therapist can lead the patient's attention away from the outer world, where she may feel that achievement will be expected, and lead it to the inner world, the deep sources of emotion and creativity. The music will form an immediate bridge between the inner and outer worlds. This can be done by starting with one of Assagioli's (1965) imagination exercises such as "Climbing a Mountain" or "Watching a Cave Mouth in the Jungle." I begin by asking the patient to imagine the scene and just give some indication of the feeling about what she is imagining on the instruments. When she discovers that her tentative taps and tones turn into a strange but satisfying kind of music with the therapist's accompaniment, she is led to play more freely and with pleasure.

For example, a schizophrenic man of 28, who had a degree in psychology and felt he knew more than the therapists, (which he surely did in some areas), was feeling that there was a quick and easy way out of his illness and hospital stay. Asked to imagine a Mountain Climb, he banged away on the drums and cymbal and said afterwards that he went up the mountain in a fast sports car and reached the top in no time. In doing this he was not only showing contempt for his analytical music therapy but also indicating his unwillingness to face the hard work that we might have to do on the depressive aspects of his condition. But the strength of his feelings brought out the musical expression with ease.

As soon as the link between phantasy, emotion and music is forged, the patient's attention is engaged, and the technique is established without self-consciousness or difficulty. When the patient's recorded music, together with the therapist's piano part, is played back, the patient will be intrigued by this experience and will then tolerate more external awareness and, amazingly enough, often be able to link the inner with the outer by pointing out the very moment of the linking of her musical sound and her inner experience.

Sometimes, instead of doing the imagination exercise, some situation from the material presented by the patient will be explored. For example, the well-educated, hysterical patient of 54, mentioned earlier, said she saw herself as a figure split in half from head to toe and being half black (on the left) and half white. The black half contained all her unused potential and the white half was a fragmented, whispy, almost transparent half which carried out the routine office jobs. We explored these two halves in music and she felt that something was sitting on the head of the white half, suppressing her, not allowing her to be whole self. It was an intriguing beginning.

A patient may show a quite different side of herself in musical expression from when she is talking before and after playing. The therapist will hold both aspects of the patient and endeavour to introduce them to each other during the work. For example, a woman patient was crying and pathetic in our verbal exchange, and robust and capable on the instruments. To unite these two aspects we played some music about the pathetic child she felt herself to be and it was the robust side that played this!

It is necessary to establish a relationship with the whole person rather than certain attractive or even unattractive aspects of it. This is much easier (though sometimes more complicated) with the added tool of musical improvisation. Therefore I would recommend using the music in the first session even if you have not finished the factual exploration of her background and have to do a bit more in the second session. I do this, partly because it gives a better view of more of the whole person, though some sub-personalities may still be hidden in the wings waiting to emerge much later; and partly because on account of some bad musical experiences, possibly at school, the patient may dread the musical part so much that she never turns up for the second session.

Lastly, although the therapist may be justifiably a little anxious in the first session with a new patient, he will help himself and the patient a great deal by being briefly aware of his own body from time to time, noting any areas of tension. The more he feels at ease in his own skin, the easier it is to detect tension in the patient and to encourage her to relax and feel at ease in this new relationship.

<u>PATIENT QUESTIONNAIRE</u>

NAME:

ADDRESS:

TELEPHONE:

DATE: *AGE:*   *BIRTHDATE:*

OCCUPATION:

SPOUSE OR PARTNER:

PARTNER'S OCCUPATION:

CHILDREN:

FATHER:

MOTHER:

SIBLINGS (Names and ages):

EDUCATION:

PROBLEM:

HOW HAS PATIENT BEEN AT WORST?

DRUG USE: *ALCOHOL USE:*   *TOBACCO USE:*

SLEEPING:

EXPRESSIVE OUTLETS:

MUSICAL HISTORY:

   INSTRUMENT:

   SINGING:

   DANCING:

EXERCISES, QIGONG OR YOGA:

MEDITATION:

PSYCHIC, SPIRITUAL OR OTHER UNUSUAL EXPERIENCES:

PURPOSE IN LIFE:

SELF-EVALUATION:

DEATHS:

HOSPITALISATIONS:

OTHER THERAPIES:

THINGS I HAVEN'T ASKED:

REFERRER'S NAME AND ADDRESS:

PAYMENT ARRANGEMENT:

TERMINATION AGREEMENT:

Essay Three

The Emotional Spectrum

During my music therapy training period, it became apparent that as the work of a music therapist was to be essentially with the emotions, it was necessary for me to find some convenient way of mapping out this area of function. I thought about it deeply and finally devised the conceptual model of the emotional spectrum. The target-shaped design shown in Figure 1 was taken from Dr. Alexander Lowen's (1965) diagram of Hate surrounding a central core of Love. The placing of the seven main emotions was based on Dr. Bruno Bettelheim's (1967) study of the pathway taken by some of the autistic children in making their way back to normal function, and also the way people have broken down, or broken through, at marathon group therapy sessions.

There are, of course, many more words for emotions than those given on the spectrum, but those are compound emotions. Jealousy, for instance, is a compound of love, fear and anger. Respect is a blend of love and freeze-fear. Pride can be love of self with defensive fear. Depression can be a mixture of sorrow, guilt and freeze-fear covering up anger.

In this model, each emotion has its positive and negative aspect. The three central emotions of love, joy and peace form a triad which should be fairly evenly balanced. In some people, love is the tonic, joy the dominant and peace the mediant. In others, the tonic is joy or peace. Most people are under-expressing in one of them and need to work consciously at restoring the balance. This can be done usefully through music therapy.

The various emotions given are no more exact than at what point between 600 Mu and 500 Mu yellow turns to green. Neverthe-less they can be a useful rough guide in the therapist's work. Here is an explanation of the spectrum.

Figure 1.

Map of Emotional Territory
(Lowen, 1965)

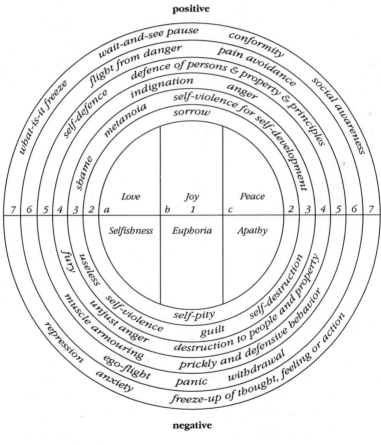

positive

negative

The Seven Main Emotions

Freeze-Fear:

+7. In animal life this is the first response of the rabbit to danger. It serves a useful purpose in humans when it enables them to think and understand what it would be best to do rather than plunging ahead recklessly.

-7. In its negative aspect freeze-fear can be seen in psychiatric illness as catatonia. As body tension it can take a less drastic form as a protection against desired but feared acts of violence or sexual appetite. It can also cause an inability to decide, act, feel or think.

Flight-Fear:

+6. In fleeing from what is harmful this is a normal, healthy response.

-6. In its negative aspect it can be heedless panic flight or flight into physical or psychiatric illness.

Defensive Fear:

+5. Any normal, useful defence of one's person, property or values comes into this category.

-5. This is the sort of behaviour which is unadaptably defensive all the time. -5 oriented characters act like alarmed hedgehogs and rhinos and are difficult to communicate with unless one remembers the vulnerability inside and addressed oneself to this. Protective compulsive ritualistic and obsessive behaviour come into this category.

Anger:

+4. This is righteous indignation and willingness to take aggression on behalf of the self or its objects and values.

-4. When anger turns into violent destruction it is negative.

Guilt:

+3. This is a useful emotion when its pain produces change for the better but it is too often combined with the negative aspect of freeze-fear and frozen solid.

-3. This is the urge to destroy the self, either quickly and dramatically or slowly through abuse of alcohol or drugs. It very often follows negative, or even positive, feelings of anger. It could be argued that it is a kind of negative anger. But it is not, as the aggression is directed inward, it has quite another quality although it can be identification with an outer persecutor who is supposed to be feeling negative anger.

Sorrow:

+2. This is a tremendously healing emotion where it is allowed to flow freely, which usually it is not. About unexpressed grief Dr. E. P. Gramlich (1968) writes, "Physical symptomatology is a common part of grief and chronic grief may be manifested by chronic physical symptoms either due to diagnosable psychosomatic conditions or ill-defined symptoms of pain and dysfunction. Parkes lists osteoarthritis, colitis, spastic colon, urticaria, migraine, asthma, bronchitis, ulcerative colitis as disease entities which may be precipitated or aggravated by a loss."

-2. Self-pity is one of the most invidious and poisoning emotions which prevents further development by its passive masochistic orientation.

Love:

+1a. This is a warm giving and receiving.

-1a. Desire is the awareness of a need, a kind of dynamic emptiness.

Joy:

+1b. This is a vitalising force expressive of delight.

-1b. Mania is used in this context as any hollow joy based on a defence against or blocking out of other emotions and is seen at its worst in the manic stage of affective disorders.

Peace:

+1c. This brings serenity to the character.

-1c. This is apathy. Not the tense inactivity of negative freeze-fear but a self-satisfied, sluggish state of being.

Recording the Emotions

The numerals on the spectrum make it a suitable way of recording the emotions expressed through different parts of the body. Imagine, for example, treating an aphasic child. His only communication will be nonverbal sounds or body expression. When making the case notes these can be neatly recorded. Draw a rough sketch of the child, a pin man will do, and then record numerically the emotions that showed themselves in the session on the appropriate parts of the body. For example little John, an undersized autistic boy of 11, only showed a -4 aggressive response in his clacking teeth for many weeks. This would be normal for a feeding baby. His hands, at this time, only showed -7 freeze-fear reaction, being clutched inwards on his chest. One week he came in when I was drinking my morning coffee. With a rush he threw himself on me and grabbed for the coffee. I was able to record his -1 and -4 response in the hands that evening. Notably enough, the -4 did not return to the teeth during that session.

In an interview a client may be responsive and smiling but expressing -7 with her legs and hands, and the freeze-fear may be a cover for her -4 in the hands and a habitual -1a response in the legs. The possibility of recording these emotional responses in the body makes the therapist more alert to their appearance and change, and able to plot the dynamic flow of emotional expression through the body over a period of time.

As an Assessment Tool

The emotional spectrum has proved to be a useful assessment tool at a client's first interview. The therapist presents the client with the basic emotion titles written on cards and places these on the floor. It is unnecessary at this stage to explain about the negative aspects, the client may interpret them as she will. Sitting before a battery of instruments, the client, who is usually in an acute state of -7, finds it relatively easy to express this in sound. Her playing is taped and played back to her when she will usually respond with a great deal of useful information about her thoughts concerning this emotion, also special occasions on her life when she experienced it as destructive or helpful.   From there the therapist proceeds through the whole spectrum.

It is important to observe how much of her body the client involves in playing the different emotions.   For example, a young psychiatrist expressing the fears used nothing but his wrists and hands. He warmed up towards the centre of the spectrum involving his shoulders in anger and his whole back and abdomen and legs in love. In his job he was habitually used to inhibiting negative fear responses but was successful in his work and a happily married man who found full expression on loving.

Here are examples of brief notes from emotional spectrum tests on a postgraduate student and a businessman.

Freeze-fear:
>   Student: Played from above, tapped, high.
>   Businessman: Couldn't do it.

Flight-fear
>   Student: Fierce thuddy, gentle withdrawal on cymbal.
>   Businessman: Glissando on xylophone.

Defensive fear
>   Student: Very fierce
>   Businessman: Very violent.

Anger
>   Student: Rather organised and jolly.
>   Businessman: Tremendous outburst.

Guilt
>   Student: Cymbal insidious, connected to depression.
>   Businessman: Couldn't do it.

Sorrow:
>   Student: Gentle, beautiful xylophone.
>   Businessman: Thoughtful.

Love:
>   Student: Strong. 4/4 on cymbal.
>   Businessman: Couldn't do it.

Joy:
>   Student: 4/4 happy, alive
>   Businessman: Conventional rhythm

Peace:

> Student: Crescendo on cymbal.
> Businessman: Sensitive

What did it mean? The answer cannot be given exactly in words. These are clues to which the therapist responds intuitively. But a little more information may be helpful. The student had a tendency for flight into illness. Her positive use of aggression was not free and was subsequently successfully developed through music therapy and used to her greater advantage. Too much of her personality was built around defending against being told how to be, instead of getting on with it and actually being herself. Love had been a positive experience. Guilt was negative but only very mildly.

The businessman was using his aggression to the full; he was very defended, even to the point of refusing to attempt to express emotions which he found troublesome. His flight-fear in life expressed itself in a constant whirl of activity. His playing of sorrow and peace showed that he was in touch with the more sensitive part of his psyche. After quite a number of sessions he was expressing love musically with gusto and agreeable lack of inhibition, and could accept freeze-fear and guilt as having their part in the scheme of things.

Experience in Groups

I have had interesting experiences going through the emotional spectrum with groups of psychiatric patients, each in turn playing their sound expression of the same emotion. Anger always brought out very lively emotional discharge in the listeners through laughter. They were well able to express the fears. Flight-fear provoked some amusement. Defensive fear produced a high casualty rate among instruments. Guilt produced seriousness on the whole with some sniggers and guffaws by an element which was troubled by feelings about masturbation. Most people found guilt hard to express but all talked about it interestingly afterwards. Sorrow brought on an atmosphere of intense interest and electric expectation; it seemed to be a depth of experience that all had plumbed but never spoken about freely before. There was a tense silence and rapt attention during performances. Love was found to be very difficult to express in sound but for this reason the verbal communication following performances was most enlightening. It is the effort which is most helpful, the result is less important.

After two terms of sound expression in this manner, I found that the same patients were quite expressive and fluent in making small impromptu speeches to the group describing incidents using these emotions. When we began it was difficult to provoke more than a monosyllable or short sentence in response to a question.

Other Uses

It can be useful for the music therapy student to practise studying emotional patterns by recording the emotions of a character in any novel which she is reading, then comparing the character's pattern with her own. A church group co-operated in making an emotional spectrum plotting of the recorded expressions of the emotions of Jesus in one gospel. It was interesting to see how many +4 notations there were in spite of the popular "meek and mild" image.

Essay Four

Techniques for Probing the Conscious

What are AMT Techniques?

An analytical music therapy technique is a particular focus for emotional investigation through music which the therapist uses with a client. The emotional inner territory is so vast and chaotic that it can be a help to both client and therapist to let their minds create and hold a certain focal structure. These techniques can, of course, be used by ordinary music therapists but it may be more difficult for them to interpret their client's unconscious symbolism without projecting unrealised parts of themselves on to it, and they will probably work more confidently by using the material at a more conscious and matter-of-fact level. Such techniques as are described in this essay and the following two have been devised, or adapted, to answer necessities arising within genuine therapeutic situations. New situations will always arise and I trust that their demands will be met by the creativity of future analytical music therapists. Meanwhile these are most of the techniques in current use.

Why use one rather than another?

When he has experienced and experimented with all these techniques in his Intertherapy training sessions, the analytical music therapist will begin to have the feeling of which technique is called for at any particular point in the therapy. Perhaps the client is blocked at a deeper level and needs to work with symbols, dreams and images; perhaps she needs help in loosening a conflict knot through the Splitting technique or perhaps she needs to find out what internal fear is holding her back from taking her next step forward in reality with a Reality Rehearsal technique. As the client talks, some kind of picture of her internal situation will develop in the therapist's mind. Something will cry out for investigation. If nothing does, then it might be the moment to see what is going on beneath the surface with one of the Guided Imagery techniques.

How many are used in one session?

This will depend on many factors: how affected the client is by her music, how much insight she can take, whether she is using words as a way of avoiding music, or music as a way of hiding from interpretation and discussion. Sometimes a whole session goes by without the therapist having been able to persuade the client to play a note and sometimes there will be four or five long improvisations with scarcely a word spoken. For the kind of client who spins out the first three-quarters of an hour with defensive chatter, an immediate free improvisation, lasting about ten minutes, is recommended. In this way, the defence is bypassed, genuine emotions are expressed, the therapist has some idea of her true feelings and has something real to relate to during the next part of the session. As clients get to know the techniques, they often cooperate usefully by asking to explore a feeling, relationship, or problem area with a certain technique. Of course, they also sometimes do this to put off the moment when they have to tell the therapist the answer which they already know and are unhappy about facing. But by this time the therapeutic couple know one another.

The Holding Technique

This technique is also sometimes called "containing." Its purpose is to allow the client to fully experience her emotion right through to its climax through emotional sound expression while being held emotionally by the musical matrix of the therapist. It is the musical equivalent of the small child going through a tantrum, heartbroken sobbing, or transports of wild delight while being safely and lovingly held and guarded by her parent. This diminishes the fear of disintegration under high emotional stress, gives the emotion the chance to evolve into something different, and dissipates enough bound energy to allow the client to think more and feel less about the subject.

The therapist must create a safe container for the client's expression by his music. It must not be a constricting container which forbids full expression. At no time should her expression exceed his so that she gets the feeling that she is having the burden of carrying him along. On the other hand his expression must not be so violent before she is ready to express her feelings as to shock her back into non-expression. If it is just right the client will probably be oblivious of it, but if it is wrong she will be uneasy and feel "let down" or constricted. During conversation, the therapist may be aware of the emotional possibilities of the matter to be investigated and, at the start, he will let the client lead, then be a little ahead in expression, urging her on to the height of the emotional experience. Having achieved this she may be fully contained but running wild in the situation unable to make the turn. His task then is gently to bring her back, and this is done by changing to tonal music and containing the frenzy in strong major common chords; then she can feel that her excitement has a place in the harmony of life and has not damaged the environment.

It is important for the therapist to cease playing the very moment the client does so and let her expression at once flow freely into words. Again the therapist is the container. This time the emotion will be expressed in a less dynamic and more concrete way and there may be an attempt to examine the reasons for the feelings after the experience has been clarified. If the mood being contained is one of sadness or mysterious peace, the client may want to remain silent. But the therapist's close attention and willing reception of this silence is also a kind of containment. He can turn an intending blocking silence into the most intimate shared experience by his receptivity and holding of the relationship. Such moments can be most pregnant and fruitful for the client when she realises that her punitive act of withholding communication is not being reciprocated, that she is not blocked out of anything but, on the contrary, while lovingly held, is being allowed to reach down and bring something up out of herself, taking as much time as she needs to do this.

The musical containing experience can be extremely taxing to the therapist. It is unwise to undertake this if the therapist has not really been through the full gamut of his own passions. Even so I can remember one particular session which almost split my mind and left my limbs so shaky that I found it quite difficult to become sufficiently composed to play the violin on the ward which I had to go to afterwards. I may say that this was a peak violent experience for the client, too. After that session things were more manageable for both of us.

Example 1

A woman of 33 came to the session terribly tense and said she was rejecting her husband sexually and blocking out the words of the consultant psychotherapist in her group meeting. After four attempts which she foiled with conversational gambits, we improvised "Rejection." She drummed with frenzied energy and determination for a long time only stopping when she had to gasp, "Gosh, my arms ache!" She was very much more relaxed following this and could then freely discuss who she felt had rejected her in the past.

Example 2

A woman of 32 talked about life being humdrum. We improvised "Everyday" and she played a brief piece in sad beats. We tried "Adventure" which was played rather timidly on a maraca, tambourine and drum but her vivid fantasy of having lots of money, new clothes, hair done every day and visits to "cafes dansants" was the start of a more adventurous real life pattern, and at the same time she found more pleasure in mothering her children.

Example 3

A man of 33 in his second month of weekly therapy wanted to explore his feelings of hope and despair about his illness. Twice he let the hopeful feelings be overcome and then the two feelings went into a terrible battle and he felt sleepy and "dropped away." This sleepy feeling was his subsequent reaction to the emotional awareness of strong feelings in conflict in himself and in the following week he frequently felt the "dropping away" sensation but took courage form the knowledge that it was part of his battle for health.

The Splitting Technique

The splitting technique is especially useful when the client has projected part of herself on to another character and, in doing so, has lost the emotion invested in this person. Let us take the example of

Grace, a timid, well-brought-up young woman, unacquainted with her own deeper feelings, and who unconsciously resents her landlady Mrs. Plum's interference with her life. Not wanting to face her own anger, she projects it on to Mrs. Plum whose actions then become coloured by Grace's anger. Grace comes to treatment in terror of this woman. By improvising as herself (Grace) while the therapist plays angry Mrs. Plum, and then playing Mrs. Plum while the therapist plays the victimised Grace, Grace has a chance to get in touch with her own anger over the situation and, with its protection as a consciously owned force, Grace can come to feel less threatened by Mrs. Plum, being now faced with this lady's real anger only and not her own projected unconscious anger ricocheting back at her as well. This is an oversimplified example, as these things take time to work through and understand. But perhaps this will at least explain the principle behind this technique.

Another use of this technique is for conflict situations where all the energy is being held in maintaining the status quo and nothing appears to be happening, but at the same time the client is quite exhausted and has difficulty in getting anything done. In this version, the client gives a word picture of her feelings about both sides of the conflict and then the music therapist starts off rigorously in the character of one person or idea. After a time it is useful to let the music become a duet, a mixing together of these opposed forces. When the client breaks off before this point, a third improvisation can be done having both titles and being carried out more on the lines of the holding technique.

Example 1

Barbara is a young wife and mother with obsessional traits. She has a violent fear and hatred of her sister Rose. I played her civilised self and she played Rose with tremendous excitement and energy. Then I was "the wild, uncontrollable Rose," and she played a two-semi-quaver and a quaver ostinato with a sforzando when she could hardly bear the excitement. Barbara could hardly resist joining my wild Rose music. Following this session she gradually began to own her own wild feelings about Rose and resist her intrusions in reality---a little unmanageably at first. Her tight, doll-like expression relaxed and she was able for the first time to show affection to her little daughter who had the same hair colouring as Rose.

Example 2

Thelma, a young office worker, had troubles over suicidal feelings. We were splitting "Chaos" and "Punishment." It was difficult to work with Thelma as she always wanted to break off relationships, life, therapy. I played "Chaos" very wildly, she rattled a maraca a little as "Punishment" and then stopped and somehow mentally froze me out. It was impossible to continue playing. She succeeded in giving me the breaking off feeling completely. This session was followed by her repeating the experience within a sexual relationship. She just got out of bed and walked out of her boyfriend's flat in the middle of the night after engaging in sexual intercourse without herself experiencing orgasm. Our subsequent examination of her fear of any kind of natural or emotional climax was very useful.

Example 3

Thelma again, prior to going abroad to work, had mixed feelings about leaving her unenthusiastic widowed mother, and was frightened that her own enthusiasm would suddenly vanish. She played herself as being sad while I played "Bright Mother." Thelma's music got more and more angry. Then I was "Sad Mother" and she was "Enthusiastic Thelma." The mother's sadness made her feel guilty, so much so that she stopped. This was the danger then. By thinking the whole idea through and making a plan of action she gained enough confidence to keep up her enthusiasm and carry out her plan.

Example 4

A university student, Eva, wanted to explore with me her unequal relationship experiences. I started by being "Doormat" while she played being "Dominant;" but rather than concentrating on her own expression, she tried to provoke me all the time. She said that she thought that if I did last out then she would have to be "Doormat." Next I was "Doormat," but I left spaces for her to answer back musically but she never did. Next I made a long decrescendo to see when she would dare to reverse roles. At my pianissimo she was even more pianissimo, and then when I reached her level of softness suddenly, right at the end, she did assert herself. Following this, she felt able to resist her tutor's efforts to make her take up work at a "suitable" school whose principles she disbelieved in, and to risk looking for a position in which she would feel happy and honest.

Investigation of Emotional Investment

This technique is used in cases where words seem to lead you round and round in a circle and you get nowhere. I have found it a very good method of comparing a client's feelings about the marriage partner and another person who has become irresistibly attractive. The client and therapist together improvise with the title of the two characters one after the other, the therapist using the Holding technique. But here the therapist is also a very sensitive accompanist and most of all a listener. He should not give way to any countertransference feelings at all, only accompany the phenomenal sounds and then listen to what is said about the two characters and compare this with the sound pictures. It is best not to play back this recording to the client as she will be very defended against the truth at this stage, but it can be taken as the basis of work in the future. This technique can also be useful when a little verbal phrase pops up again and again obviously loaded with special meaning and emotion. In this case the therapist will use countertransference feelings as in the Holding technique.

Example 1

Beryl was a young wife with two children; her marriage had deteriorated until it was a sharing of child rearing, home and money. But she had met Oliver, an older man who doted on her, visited her daily in hospital (unlike her husband), idealised her, wrote her romantic letters telling her that he would wait until her children were grown up. He was totally undemanding sexually. The improvisation on Oliver showed a very rhythmic, gentle feeling almost like rocking a cradle. The improvisation on the husband was arhythmic, dynamic with many different kinds of expression. I put my money on the legal relationship. The next week, on an impulse, Beryl went out to visit Oliver without warning and found him in bed with another woman. The marriage took a turn for the better. Here her words had convinced me that her marriage was dead and Oliver a kind, unselfish possible replacement. But her music said otherwise.

Example 2

Kathleen, 33, with three children, was wildly in love with Ian and unable to have any feelings for her husband but those of a child. We improvised "Affair" but there was not much emotional engagement. When we played "Marriage" (meaning her present marriage) there was much more depth, a feeling of contentment which she said was in the marriage and with the children. Kathleen battled through all these feelings, another woman conveniently went off with Ian, and she and her husband subsequently came to a much better understanding. Later, this woman having abandoned Ian, Kathleen had a very brief affair with him but returned with a deeper commitment to her husband.

Example 3

Vera, 30, was complaining of her fear of travelling in buses, especially waiting at the stops. We improvised "Waiting," the music was rather subdued but played on every instrument there. Her inner experience was of waiting, being faint, getting on the bus, fainting, not being able to visit her mother but having to be taken back to her husband. This led to several sessions of sorting out feelings about her father and husband. Some time later she was coming to the sessions quite confidently by bus.

Entering into Somatic Communication

Sometimes physical symptoms are messages telling you that you have wrenched a muscle and must be careful how you move; sometimes they are communications about emotion which has been bypassed by conscious experience, or "organ-jargon." On the latter case they can be stubbornly resistant to the usually helpful remedies. If the client can let the therapist play "Her" while she fully puts herself into being the symptoms, she can often get in touch with the by-passed emotion and, because of the tension released in the music, allow herself to experience it. When she does it may be very painful indeed. Such mechanisms are not in use for nothing. But what one experiences one can talk about, think about and work on; when the emotion is hidden one is helpless. Sometimes, too, genuinely organic symptoms are also the carriers of communications about by-passed feelings and this can make them more difficult to tolerate and treat.

Example 1

Vera (see Example 3 on the previous page) came to her session looking rather depressed. She had a severe headache following a row with her husband. She played the "Headache" and I was her, it was a nice bit of chamber music. During this music she felt very angry indeed. Then we reversed it and she was herself as patient victim, feeling just the headache. She had a great deal of guilt about her aggression, and if she expressed any she always turned the residue against herself. Earlier this had been expressed by taking overdoses of sleeping pills; the headaches were, in this case and in many others, a beginning of being able to contain and transmute these feelings more constructively.

Example 2

Ian, 32, was having trouble coping with his partially released aggression and was sometimes experiencing pains in his neck and shoulders and a "wandering" feeling in his head. On being the "Wandering," he played with tremendous force, hammering the xylophone keys till they leapt off their pegs; then when he heard the playback he found that he got the pains and his hands were gripping the divan where he lay, the knuckles white with tension. He subsequently adopted a more interested, experimental approach to his various symptoms, not feeling so much of a helpless victim, and a short while later, without outside coercion, willingly took on more challenging work.

Postscript

All the clients and patients in these examples were coming for music therapy sessions over a period of time for quite serious disturbances. These were not one-session treatments.

With regard to the patients in hospital no one can be sure whether it is the chemotherapy, group psychotherapy, individual psychotherapy, art therapy, music therapy, occupational therapy, industrial therapy, the fellow patients, the nursing, the cooking, the chaplain, time the healer, or what that helps most. I find it a good rule to warmly congratulate all my colleagues for any successes with mutual patients which I think that I may have helped with. What one sees in one's own sessions one is sure about but it is only part of the whole picture that reveals itself when the team meet. Everyone has a part to play and no one should be made to feel unimportant.

Essay Five

Techniques for Accessing the Unconscious

Using Symbols

The techniques described in Essay Four were all suitable for investigating conditions of which both the therapist and client were fully aware. They are perhaps the easiest for the lay reader to understand but they are not by any means the first techniques to be applied in treatment. Too often clients present the conscious mind in a state of painful aridity, due to the lack of any creative and fruitful relationship with the unconscious. They never dream, they say, or if they do, their dreams are quite meaningless and immediately forgotten. The inner geography is a stony, pessimistic desert, the season a perpetual winter. Their outer life reflects this picture. This is the time for using symbols.

Symbols are accumulators and transformers of psychic energy. They have the relationship to ideas and action that an iceberg has to a waterfall. Using them, the therapist is dealing with the transformation of force. Normally this can be very tricky but the music therapist has this unique lightning conductor: the tapping off of the surplus emotional dynamism through shared sound expression. It is not the psychic energy that turns to glowing cheeks, shining eyes, humming nerves through the body, and laughter, passion or tears, that is dangerous. It is the cold, frantic denial of emotion that causes horrible splits in the mind and leaks out into strange ideas, bodiless voices and chill moonlit inner landscapes.

At the beginning of treatment then, there is often this need for a loosening-up process whereby the unconscious can be allowed to fertilise the conscious mind. At this time the client's symbols will tell the therapist the things which she cannot herself say, simply because she is not aware of them. But once expressed and experienced they have an effect on her. They have their own most convincing reality which is often felt to add a richness and an added dimension to an otherwise sterile inner life. They also have a purpose in outer reality, and it is the therapist's task to create a bride from the manifest symbol to its meaningful expression in outer reality. If this is not done the client can get drawn inwards---almost like a drug addict is---enjoying the images but shrugging off all responsibility as to the meaning and purpose of their translation into everyday life and work and endeavour. In this way, far from transmuting her energy into her individual conscious life, her little remaining energy will seep back into the inner life to try to find satisfaction there. For this reason the analytical music therapist will encourage clients working with symbols to "earth," or "concretise" the energy through as many modalities as possible. For example, first will come the inner realisation accompanied by the musical expression. This will be followed by a description of the symbol in words with details about the client's feelings and physical sensations experienced during the musical expression. Then the client may draw with coloured crayons or paint, however crudely, the symbol when she gets home and once again different attributes and meanings will be discovered. These may then be the basis for another musical investigation at a more conscious level. In this way the energy will be safely transformed and all the time the meaning for outer life will be discussed.

Two kinds of client are very difficult to work with in this way. One is the very extraverted client who cannot see beneath the surface of anything and has no awareness of the noumenal side of life. If her defences can be gently eased she may benefit greatly from the use of these techniques. The other is the client who is too introverted and needs firmer hold on reality through a well-made bridge from unconscious to conscious and the growing willingness to be responsible for the outer expression, through sound expression of inner realisations. The immediate tapping off of the emotion through sound expression held in the therapist's music greatly reduces any possible danger of "flooding" by the unconscious. Music therapists vary in their ability to enable clients to realise these inner images and what one client can experience with one therapist she may be quite unable to experience with another.

Guided Imagery

These techniques have been adapted from some examples given in Dr. Robert Assagioli's book Psychosynthesis (1965). The first three are very useful early on in treatment and the fourth can be useful throughout. The client should be told what scene to conjure up but not to think about what will happen. "Just see the scene and start playing, let anything happen but keep contact with me through your sound expression," is roughly what she is told. Some clients find it hard to visualise anything at all before their music has reduced some of their emotional pressure. They can be given a preliminary Holding exercise on Anxiety or Fear to reduce tension. Others have a very impressive experience and break off in fright. They should be encouraged to go back to the scene and come to some kind of conclusion. This is usually reassuring to them. The therapist's musical technique will be as in Holding and his countertransference expression can be of the greatest possible assistance to the client's inner realisations.

The Cave Mouth

The client imagines that she is standing hidden behind a tree in a forest clearing watching the mouth of a cave. As she watches, something emerges. The forms that emerge are usually symbolised projections of suppressed or undeveloped areas of the client's responsibility. They can be understood as pre-verbal images. *Plato - The Cave -*

Example 1

A young woman of 32 with depressions, making a very feeble contribution in marital and maternal roles, improvised with lively music and experienced going into the cave, being attacked by bats, which she fought and then found a pirate's treasure of coins and jewels. Being encouraged to go back and get it out she experienced going to get help, bringing the treasure home and having a party. In her case the black bats of angry depression had prevented her from using her true inner wealth. The step of "going to get help" was a significant one which was later acted out in useful ways during her treatment period.

Example 2

A university student, with a feeling of a splitting between her inner and outer self, also entered a cave which was wet and cold and there was a "sinister lurking" feeling and a sensation that the walls would fall in. The music was very sensitive and expressive. This was, in her case, tied up with the fear of a kind of implosion with no protective affirmative radiation from a true centre of being. It gave an indication of how to proceed by setting out to help her find, and play from, this centre.

Example 3

A young wife and mother with hysterical suicidal impulses saw a lion come out of the cave and she fought it again and again until at last her steady beat at the end showed that she had won. She slowly began to make the psychiatrists and other attackable persons into lions for fighting instead of turning all this feeling against herself. Later on situations to be conquered were lions.

Ascending a Mountain

In this technique the client imagines that she is climbing a mountain and is asked afterwards to report on such details as the climate, the terrain, the size of the mountain, view from the top if reached, her apparel and any obstacles in the way of the ascent. The mountain is the measure of aspiration in life and the obstacles inner or outer hindrances.

Example 1

A man of 49, a taxi-driver, showed little emotion in his playing. He said he saw the mountain, it was not more than a green hill really and he thought why should he bother to climb it anyway, he would go for a walk in the sunshine instead. This was typical of his attitude to life which was to try to get some fleeting sensual pleasure out of his days while life lasted, without regarding the cumulative results of his actions or other possible sources of satisfaction which might be more lasting. He was a very unhappy man under the mask of a happy-go-lucky fellow and grossly obese.

Example 2

A university student with identity problems felt expansion as she climbed to the top of an English mountain. We discussed why it was such a small one. She tried another, abroad. As she toiled up I experienced overwhelming depression by countertransference and then she stopped and said she could not go on, it was grey and hard and cold and lonely. She spoke of her two siblings, one (whom she rather despised) who had settled for a safe, routine job, and the other (her ideal), who was so dedicated and earnest about his work that it seemed to leave no room for feelings and pleasant side alleys. We were able to look at other possible models and she subsequently adopted a much more creative and individual approach to her own career and talents.

Example 3

A young man of 29 had an immature personality. His playing was extremely sensitive, using the drum and cymbal at first alternately and then together with some excitement and with responsive musical interplay with the therapist. There was no feeling of form and it went on so long that finally I had to end it. He said that he had imagined himself toiling up a mountain with snow and blizzards raging all around him and then had just been lost in the music. His lone parent had died when he was 16 and he had lived with relatives and taken various jobs, but had broken them all off or been asked to leave through quarrelling with his work-mates. One could say that he had a life pattern of losing his aspirational aim through getting lost in the music of the emotional interplay.

Example 4

A young woman with compulsive suicidal impulses did some of the most solid and rhythmic drumming that I had ever heard from her in climbing the mountain. She reached the top and said it was marvelous that she had struggled up there in spite of all her slipping back. This was a pattern of effort and achievement that we often looked back on through the next year of just that kind of progress.

The Pool in the Meadow

The client imagines that she enters a meadow and goes and looks into a pool in the far left corner to see what emerges or what she can see in the pool. This exercise usually shows disturbances in the sexual sphere in the form of repressive or regressive tendencies of the personality.

Example 1

A woman of 32, wife and mother, who was frigid, entered the meadow going past cows and horses and looked into the pool, on which there were ducks, and saw her own reflection which she said she disliked. This brought up some interesting discussion about this bad feeling concerning her image and how embarrassed she had been as a girl at the arrival of her ample bosom. Her painting of this scene led to further improvisations and pictures and there was a subsequent amelioration of her condition.

The Door in the High Wall

This technique aims at releasing, in pre-verbal imagery, symbols clustered round any idea which is felt to need investigation. The client imagines a long, high wall in which there is a door marked with the matter of the enquiry, such as: "Fear," "Love," "Why..." The client imagines that she goes through the door and notices what is on the other side. Sometimes out of the jumble of images a feeling of certainty and great peace emerges.

Example 1

A woman in her forties was experiencing very painful and

time-resonating jealousy. (A time-resonating emotional experience is one which is loaded with a disproportionate amount of feeling from an event in the past, the impact of which was unexpressed or possibly unacknowledged at that time). The door marked "Jealousy" turned into a bird cage with a green eagle's head pecking at its own throat and then a huge claw attacking its breast. The cage faded into green and blue clouds with sudden red points. "Like nipples which can only feed one at a time," she said. Then there was a veiled moon and a white flame, and "a feeling that the moon cannot accept the sun's light because of the green clouds." She was asked to become the moon and said, "A beautiful, mysterious Venus was locked in the moon and she whispered a world of marvelous feminine secrets to me." As the bird, she said, "I was attacked instantly by terrible feelings in the throat and chest while I played on the guiro and screamed raucously and then suddenly thought, 'That is what I am doing to K' (the object of jealousy) and felt ashamed." She was profoundly moved by this experience and subsequently battled hard to let calm thought into this area of painful feelings and potentially spiteful action.

Myths

This is a technique which I have not found it necessary to use as yet in individual therapy. It is indicated where the client feels that directly personal imagery and emotion are in some way threatening. The therapist will read out a simplified version of a myth or fairy tale such as the legend of Orpheus or Cinderella, and using the Holding technique they will improvise together, imagining each scene. The personal deviations from, and the details added to, the original story can be used fruitfully in discussion, and the musical expression and relationship will tell the therapist something about the feelings which the client so much wanted to hide from him.

Intracommunication

This is a method for working on dreams. All contents of normal dreams can be thought of as parts of the dreamer split off and put temporarily outside her awareness to be looked at. The therapist notes down the client's dream or dream fragment with each noun having a separate line and number. The client first gives associations to each item then enters them in turn and speaks as if she were they. Parts of the dream can then be improvised on and items which did not meet or confront one another in the dream can communicate as in the Splitting technique. The client is then encouraged to find the meaning of the dream for her real-life situation. Whether or not a person believes that dreams do have a purpose, the search for meaning is, in itself, a valuable exercise and brings up a great deal of useful material to work on.

Example 1

With a phobic woman of 38, wife. mother and part-time employee, I worked on the following dream during her second month of therapy. The associations are in brackets and the intracommunication in quotes. The dream went like this: she was sitting on a box of dead people (grey tin box) "Open the lid;" in a ruined building with water running down the walls (mother is a ruin, frightening, dark, dank walls) "This is you;" she was with someone, (she quite liked it) "What's she doing sitting on my box?", who said, "Let's open it." In the box were four bodies face down (I wanted to sit on the lid to suffocate them, they were not quite dead) "I'm beautiful," "I'm warm and secure," "I'm dead," "I'll leave her;" the last one, a man in a brown suit (dull, nondescript, husband?) walked away carrying with him a small deed box "I'm taking the soul with me." We improvised a Splitting of the people sitting on the box: the Suffocators and the people being suffocated. As Suffocator she felt just heavy and dull with slow thudding drum beats. Being suffocated, she played with the liveliest drum and cymbal crashes I had heard from her, feeling vehemently, "I won't be suffocated!" There were memories, when we talked afterwards, of being shut in her room at two, a feeling that through her phobia her creative side was being suffocated and the keen realisation of both the energy and will for life in this part of her as well as the fear of exposure and challenge of growth. Some time later she told me of a secret suitcase full of stories which she had written which no one except her husband had ever seen.

Dream Resolution

In this exercise the client goes back and finds, in an improvisation, another ending to the kind of unsatisfactory or frightening dream from which one wakes in a state of disturbance or haunted feeling which can last for days, weeks or even years. It is a most reassuring experience, rather like tidying a room internally. The only recorded example which I have is unfortunately quite unfit for this kind of publication.

Shells, Stones, Sand and Sounds

Sand play

This technique can have an almost hypnotically calming effect or, occasionally, one of extreme irritation. It is based on the experience of sitting on the seashore idly arranging shells to the sound of the sea. The client sits by the chime bars with a tray of white sand and a bowl of shells and stones, and while the therapist answers her on the xylophone and cymbal (with wire brush only) she places a shell (or stone) on to the sand. She then repeats this process until she has had enough. She is not told to have any conscious focus, just to do it. But this idle meaninglessness can bring out the deepest meaning. Very often a client who is blocking expression in one modality cannot resist allowing herself an outlet through another.

Example 1

A woman in her forties, experiencing "emptiness", started by playing small steps up and down the scale getting stronger and stronger. As I played angrily on the cymbal responding to counter-transference, she sought deeper tones and played first "Killing" the notes (stopping the vibration with the beater) and then letting them sing. She took a long time over it. With shells she made two neat families of six at the bottom right hand corner and five further up. Afterwards she talked about her love of "killing people off." There were six in her parents' family, then the father died leaving five.

Example 2

Another woman, a busy professional with a family, made a harmonious design filling the whole tray and played measured tones. She felt it was a marvelous "held" feeling, like being a child who is helped but not interfered with by an adult in conversation. A satisfying nonverbal experience like this does not always call for explanation and investigation; it can be its own good reason for being.

Essay Six

Techniques for Ego-Strengthening

Most of the techniques described in this essay are designed to keep the ego much more firmly in control of matters than those in the last essay. The first three techniques are suitable for later treatment when the loosening up of the access of the unconscious has done its work and there is a greater need for tightening up and achieving conscious control and creativity in external reality.

Reality Rehearsal

When the client has reached a point of decision as to a direction to be taken in external life, she is ready for a reality rehearsal. The purpose of this technique is to raise, face, and eventually overcome or come to terms with all those inner fears, anxieties, ambivalences and negative and destructive urges which wait beside the pathway to the desired aim. Having been thus faced and at least partially overcome, they are not likely to surprise and overwhelm her when she really sets out for the interview, to the altar, to the examination or whatever the situation is, nor will they be so likely to wait for her in the small hours alone later on. Certain occult schools talk about this psychological reality as the "Dweller on the threshold" who must be reckoned with before certain pathways can be entered. The saying, "No one who puts his hand to the plough and looks back is fit for the kingdom of God," could also suggest the idea of progress being impeded by something having been left behind and not dealt with at the outset.

In this technique, the client imagines that she is taking her new step, and while keeping all her expression for her sense of purpose and endeavour, she allows herself to experience inwardly any fears and negative urges which may arise, afterwards sharing these verbally with the therapist and possibly examining them musically too. It is a well known phenomenon that at the end of treatment or psychoanalysis there can be a return of symptoms as a kind of "Dweller at the Gateway" of the new independent life. This technique goes to meet this phenomenon in a creative, constructive way just as the youth in the fairy story took food to appease the watchdogs.

Example 1

A young wife of 26, with young children was in a floundering marriage. Her husband came to ask for a reconciliation and she wanted to improvise "Making a go of it." Her playing was spasmodic, finally fading out, but she had a pleasant fantasy of painting the children's room and making love.

It is interesting to note that so many clients who can express intense emotion on the negative side (this client was remarkable for it) find it extremely difficult to invest emotion in a positive aim. This is something that has to be learnt. They imagine that the ideal will produce the emotion, as in the negative expression, whereas they must evoke and inject the expression into the idea and will its continuation. In the first case they are tapping a repressed but available source of energy and in the second they are acting as an energy producer and director, which is more difficult.

Wholeness

After all the techniques of Splitting, Holding and dipping into the great sea of the unconscious, this technique comes as quite a shock. The client plays alone, on any instrument she chooses, while the therapist listens. She is told to play as if she were perfectly whole.

Example 1

A woman of 40 said: "I sat in silence for a long while, feeling my power, almost like a god before creation. I felt my lack of balance, my dependence on some people and my vital negative resistance to others. Where was my balance? My wholeness? I felt that I had never had such total permission-to-be before and I was terrified. The therapist's calm presence held me to my endeavour. Finally I struck the gong. The responsibility was total. I played some more but all the time I felt that I was creased up in my non-wholeness of reaction and rebellion like a snail suddenly deprived of its inner-wrinkled shell. What had I gained? The potent moment of questioning. I often return to that moment in the bustle of life. It has given me a kind of secret point of growth."

Exploring Relationships

This can be done in a variety of ways: the client being the other party and letting the therapist be her as in the Splitting technique; just playing, with the partner's name as title as in Emotional Investment; or acting out different kinds of relationship musically. The emotional expression in the music seems to enable the client to receive valuable insights without the need to be told anything by the therapist. Indeed spoken words might be given at a level of understanding at which she might find the insights unassimilable.

Example 1

A man of 35 reported that his marriage was not going well but did not immediately tell that he had been having brief extramarital affairs. The therapist and client tried different ways of relating in music. First the client went his way and the therapist, as wife, went hers. Then each listened to the other while playing. Next he followed her and lastly she followed him. Afterwards he said that he liked the second way of relationship best and went on to talk very freely about his life and loves. At last he came round to feeling that the main thing that he was aware of was his great need of his wife. This session had no follow-up as the client was discharged.

Example 2

A married woman, 28, with children, explored her feelings about her lover. Improvising on his name she played with an unusually steady and guarded beat saying afterwards that she had felt love, sexual feelings and happiness but had got through to the feeling that she did not really want to leave her husband and children. The affair subsequently broke up.

Example 3

A man of 32 with angry feelings at the mother who had left him when he was four was told to tell me (as Mother) in sound all the angry feelings that he had about my going and I was to state the mother's feelings back in sound. He pounded and drummed and clashed the cymbals with enormous fierceness and then the whole feeling flowed so beautifully in to words beginning, "I feel angry and bitter..." and carrying on a whole argument without stopping for seven minutes.

Affirmations

Music therapy is not all storm and stress. There are moments of joy and peace in life which even in memory have a revivifying effect on the body through the imagination. Sometimes a client can experience a resurgence of hope and faith through getting in touch with these experiences.

Example 1

A married woman, 26, took the title "The Happiest Moment in My Life" and went back three years to the time when her baby was born. Although referred to the therapist by the psychiatrist as "lacking in confidence" she had the courage to choose to play the piano for this improvisation leaving the therapist the other instruments, and she played really beautiful music. Afterwards, describing the experience, the therapist said that her eyes shone with happiness and she looked quite radiant. The depression was momentarily banished.

Sub-verbal Communication

This technique consists of the therapeutic couple just playing without titles or focus but sometimes with a time limit of five, ten or twenty minutes. It can be a very powerful experience, even a trainee music therapist who had been through analysis said, "One is not prepared for what may come up." I use this technique when embarrassment is blocking the client's real feelings through words, when I feel that there is some difficulty in expression arising from negative or positive transference feelings or when I feel that the client is thoroughly dried out with words.

Example 1

The client was a student unable to find her centre. We played for ten minutes---perhaps we did have an unspoken title: "From the Centre"---her mechanical playing became more and more secure and then louder and then very sensitive and real as we ended. The client became aware of these changes towards a more inner-directed (centrifugal) playing.

Example 2

A married woman of 35, with children, was splitting her transference between me, as good therapist, and a former therapist, as bad. With no title or focus we played for ten minutes. She gradually expressed more and more fierce feelings on the cymbal and drum which I answered, and then at the end she expressed great tenderness. This gave us some really fierce and tender feelings within the session to talk about and it was followed by more fury in some correspondence to me later on, of which we were able to make good use in a subsequent session. She began to tolerate ambivalent feelings towards one person.

Patterns of Significance

This technique is used to discover the inner pattern and feelings surrounding significant events in life. It is particularly useful for clients in the second half of life. The main events used as titles so far have been Death, Birth, Giving Birth and Marriage. The improvisation on "Death" can cover physical death, losing a job or a limb, experiencing loss of any kind. "Birth" can be one's physical birth, birth into the adult world, any kind of initiation of entry into a new job or phase of life. "Giving Birth" may be an ordinary labour, the birth of a work of art or idea, and "Marriage" can be two people uniting as man and wife, two people in any complementary working relationship or the creative and receptive Yin-Yang powers coming together in fertile embrace in the developing psyche.

The results of this technique are in the form of feelings and yet they can have the strangely moving quality of a reality more persuasive than all the outer events of Monday to Sunday. The therapist plays as in the Holding technique.

Example 1

An unmarried woman of 50 improvised "Marriage." There was before her a valley like a rocky, bronze chalice in which there were stony hollows echoing one to the other, and she thought of the words, "Deep calling unto deep." There was a feeling of great width and no sense of nearness, closeness or anything personal. By counter-transference the therapist had the intuition to play these deep sounds. When they finished the therapist suggested that the great bowl could be her late mother's marriage and all her relationships might have been held within this. The client was told to go back and break up the valley. She felt very apprehensive about this when she started but she went at it with a will and as the drum boomed and cymbals clashed, gods and goddesses were hurled among the rocks as the valley broke up. Next there were dark green shoots of grass and a patch of pure white sand (possibly male and female symbols). She felt rather uneasy at this and then felt that she was stuck. As we played on she saw a trickle of water get bigger and bigger until it became a fountain in whose bubbling waters she bathed with a feeling of deep satisfaction. There was much to discuss and think about from this improvisation.

Example 2

A teacher of 32 played an improvisation "Giving Birth." His playing was very delicate at the beginning when he had the feeling of something growing bigger and bigger inside him. With heavy drum beats he felt that it had come out but that it was difficult to detach himself from it. The final music expressed his terrible sadness because he felt that he had lost something. He said, "It was all very selfish, I tried to think it was succeeding and being happy in its success but there was this undercurrent of deep sadness." We were then able to discuss how this resembled his feelings about letting his able pupils go out into the world when their studies were finished.

Suicide

This technique is used to allow clients (or more often patients) who want to kill themselves, to go through the feelings about such an experience. However, they are also asked, whatever they believe, to imagine for the sake of the exercise, that they have not gone out like a light but remain conscious, though invisible, and go and revisit their family and friends without, however, being able to speak to them or touch them. It is not a technique that is used lightly and never (outside the Intertherapy) unless the patient seriously brings up her wish for death by her own hand.

Example 1

This is an example of the use of this technique in an emergency together with other techniques. A wife, the mother of an 18-month-old child, suffering from moodswing, came to the psychodynamic movement session saying that she felt so awful that she wanted to die. It happened that she was the only patient to come to the session that day. Her face was pale and puffy and her eyes somehow veiled. We put on Indian music saying that we would all dance the feeling of wanting to withdraw. Suddenly there was a splintering crash; she had pushed the glass out of one of the windows and stood still, stunned. I examined her hands. Owing to the gauze curtains in front of the windows they were quite unscathed. She wanted to lie down so I gave her a cushion and rug and kept up two-way communication. Mr. O. came in, having swept away the glass outside and said perhaps she would really let us feel her anger and pain in sound. She agreed and while Mr. O. played on the piano she raged on the drum and cymbal, her face contorted with rage and dark hair flying. When she had finished she said she would have to be locked up now. "If you think so, go and tell the Sister. You are grown up," I said. She replied that she didn't feel it. Mr. O. asked her to play being the age she felt. "About three," she said starting to play in a very stilted way and getting gradually wilder and wilder and crashing on the cymbal. I asked her about her brothers and sisters. She had one brother, he was 18 months old when she was three, the same age as her own child whom she dared not look after. It looked like a displacement of her early jealousy. She then improvised on a suicide by being run over by a train. It was very wild and she stopped when she was dead saying "I feel fine." That is the moment the therapist dreads so we quickly asked her to go back and visit her family. She played for some time and stopped on the point of tears saying that she loved them so but was no good to them now. Her distress was very real. She then talked perfectly coherently for some time with shining eyes, high colour and her face looking somehow thinner. Without any extra sedation she spent the rest of the day in helping sensibly with the chores. Of course she was not cured of her very severe disorder by this but she was much alleviated and it helped her to communicate in a more normal manner.

Example 2

A wife and mother in her thirties, with compulsive urges to snatch up broken glass and knives and try to cut her wrists in order to kill herself, improvised her suicide completely through. She experienced killing herself, being happy thinking, "I've done it," then finding that she was unable to communicate with her family; going to her dead relatives and discovering that "I could not talk to them because my distress at what I had done put them out of my reach," and then coming back to her family and being distraught at not being able to be seen by them. This patient also had a very serious disturbance and she was certainly not cured by this exercise but she did come to realise how much her children meant to her and their photo, which she would hold in her hands, helped her to withstand these impulses many times.

Programmed Regression

During periods of emotional disturbance people very often regress and live partly as if they were at an earlier age, as did the young mother in the Suicide Example 1. By making the regression conscious it is easier for them to be aware of what is happening and also to return to the present. Clients are not asked to "try to remember being six" (or whatever the desired age is), they are simply told to be that age and start playing. This has never seemed to present them with the slightest difficulty. The emotions released are usually strong and frequently accompanied by vivid memory pictures of outer and inner events of that time. In the case of very early regression one cannot check up on the memory of the pre-verbal images but they seem to be of significance to the patients who produce them. Whether they really are images from their earliest infancy or feelings about that time one cannot know, but in going through such regression improvisation one can experience such a power of emotion, feel the being of the prescribed age so vividly, that I see no reason to imagine that there is a certain tender age earlier than which all this ceases and there is no more possible memory. This technique is useful for tapping the reservoir of the unexpressed in the past or for finding out at what age a certain fear or feeling began. The therapist uses the Holding technique or sometimes uses a Splitting technique with significant characters from the scenes remembered.

Example 1

A young married woman with children told the story of how she had found her sister in bed with her husband. When I asked what her reaction had been, she said that she had said, "Charming!", and walked out. I suggested that she relive the scene but express her real feelings about the situation with me. She drummed furiously for several minutes with wild shrieks of "Fucking bitch!".

It was not a matter of working herself up to it, the emotion came right out at once in this otherwise rather precise and controlled young woman.

Example 2

Joan, a phobic woman of 36, brought up the feeling of being let down on her birthday. We improvised on her second birthday, she used the drum and said it was "a happy little party"; the third birthday using the drum and cymbal was happy. On her fourth birthday, playing on the xylophone, she felt rather lost. It was just pre-war. Then she said that she could not remember her fifth birthday. I replied that she was not asked to remember but just be there and play. It was deep, sad music. When Joan finished she remembered that the nursery helper who had shown her all her dresses, including the one that she would have worn for the party, had been suddenly dismissed by Joan's father and Joan had felt so embarrassed. It is interesting how the music, in expressing her emotions, unblocked her memory of this baffling childhood event.

Example 3

A young wife, anxious about separation from anyone for whom she cared deeply, went back to the age of 12 when her uncle had taken her to visit her much loved dying aunt in a cancer ward. The music was quite stormy and violent with hints of panic. She had not been able to tell anyone her feelings at the time. "I just wanted to get out," she said. This battle of love and fear had been locked up for years.

Example 4

A widow with moodswing, 60 years old, went back to five minutes old. She was aware of light and bright colour, but around her and coming towards her was a shadow. This she managed to condense into the symbol of a cloaked figure---she said it was the figure of Death. In a later session she had images of Light and Darkness and their interaction. Light wanted Darkness to go away by becoming engulfed by it. Darkness wanted to accompany Light wherever it went and said it was there first. (It is interesting to note that another victim of moodswing, working with a different analytical music therapist, had had a similar figure of incredible darkness and evil which she became aware of in her "Birth" improvisation.)

Essay Seven

The Therapist-Patient Relationship

The therapist-patient relationship is a vital factor for the growth of the patient. In my view it aims to be a committed, non-grasping but holding relationship; at the same time, it is a holding back to receive the patient's projected parts of herself that she cannot yet integrate creatively and fruitfully within her psyche. It also aims to be a warm but non-demanding relationship as impersonal yet personally-expanding as sunlight.

It is not to be imagined, however, that the therapist is an immutable entity working on a malleable patient. As the patient struggles with her conflicting inner forces, she can work against the healing direction of the therapist. Her destructive projections can be taken right into the therapist's inner life where they will war against the very person who is there to help her. This notion is more active than the concept of the resistance. When a patient is battling seriously with a crisis in growth it is possible for the therapist to experience very testing levels of frustration, rage, despair and other difficult emotions. At such times he may have to learn to become aware of certain weaknesses in himself and then there can be significant growth on both sides if he rises to the challenge that this presents. For this reason it is extremely helpful for the therapist to have a good supervisor in his early years of practice.

Viktor Frankl (1963) points out that "The crucial agency in psychotherapy is not so much the method but rather the relationship between the patient and his doctor or, to use a currently popular expression, the 'encounter' between the therapist and the patient. This relationship between two persons seems to be the most significant aspect of the therapeutic process, a more important factor than any method or technique. However, we should not be disdainful of technique, for in therapy a certain degree of detachment is indispensable."

The therapist may well see his technique as being the most important curative factor, but in fact---everything that he is, everything that he has become through what he has done or thought or believed or felt throughout his life---all this affects the impact of the encounter. His unspoken attitudes to his profession speak to the patient. I quote from my book Music Therapy in Action: "Why is he doing this work? Is it for money? The status? The superior feeling of being able to help less fortunate individuals? The respectable voyeurism into the lives of others? The joy of sharing music? The intellectual interest in puzzling out patients' behaviour? The fascination in following up an unfoldment of being? The satisfaction of helping someone to extract a meaning from a meaningless situation? A feeling of love of humanity focussed on each individual at a time? Love of himself in the role of music therapist? The possibility of being able to cherish his fragile self in the client? Joy in doing battle against some of the ills of the age? The sharing of musical creativity bringing it into the reach of every client? Trying to make up for relationships in which he feels he has been very destructive?" (Priestley, 1975, p. 227).

Each one of these motives is human, valid and acceptable but if only one dominates the encounter, it may ultimately make the therapist's work lop-sided and even anti-therapeutic. These attitudes are so important to the patient that it is very much worthwhile for the trainee analytical music therapist to pay attention to his own self-development after becoming conscious of which hidden motives are influencing his work. This is the great value in discovering something about himself and his feelings and phantasies through his work in Intertherapy, which involves experiencing both the client and therapist roles under the supervision of a trained analytical therapist.

The founders of different schools of therapy have had different recommendations concerning the encounter between the therapist and patient, and it may well be possible that each accented the qualitites that were weakest in himself, taking his own strong points for granted and not finding it necessary to speak about them. This may explain why Freud wrote so passionately of the temptations offered to the therapist by the patient's transference love: "I cannot advise my colleagues too urgently to model themselves during psycho-analytical treatment on the surgeon, who puts aside all his feelings, even his human sympathy, and concentrates his mental forces on the single aim of performing the operation as skillfully as possible." (Complete Works, Volume 12, p. 115). Yet it is impossible to read his case histories without coming to the conclusion that he must have had a great depth of warmth and acceptance of the patient to allow for the free emergence of the deep material that he writes about. In fact, in the case study of the Rat Man, Freud even mentions feeding his patient on one occasion, which does not sound too much like a surgeon. A living link with him which seems to confirm my theory is that a friend went with her mother and emotionally disturbed sister to see Freud in Vienna. At first he was very much the professor, aloof and on his dignity, but later after the interviews with the three of them together and with the patient alone, he acted more like a family father. He was warm and friendly. It was as if the effort had to go into being aloof and the warmth came by itself when he had relaxed his guard.

In his book, Memories, Dreams and Reflections, Jung (1963) emphasized the importance of confronting each patient as one human being to another. We might speculate as to whether the temptation to hide true humanity behind a professional persona, or role mask, may originally have been quite strong in this Swiss pastor's son. He may have seen his father hiding behind the role of priest to protect his vulnerable humanity and decided that this did not consitute a healing relationship. Instead, he would strip himself bare of such shields and meet his patients face to face with honesty.

That he succeeded in attaining a rich and flexible humanity and not defending himself with any rigid professional persona is shown by one man and woman's impressions of him in later life after several meetings, not as patients but as interested friends. (Incidentally the two people were my parents). My father said that Jung was large-scale, both physically and mentally, he had a great sense of humour, no pomposity, a complete and a very satisfactory kind of man, very impressive. My mother said that she was impressed by him physically and superphysically. He was very warm, understanding, sympathetic, compassionate; a full, rich man, genuine, simple, strong and certain of himself. He had eyes that pierced yours with friendliness.

The American psychotherapist Carl Rogers stesses the need for the therapist's warm, positive regard towards the patient. In his book, Client-Centered Therapy, he writes: "In the emotional warmth of the relationship with the therapist, the client begins to experience a feeling of safety as he finds that whatever attitude he expresses is understood in almost the same way that he perceives it, and is accepted. He is then able to explore, for example, a vague feeling of guiltiness which he has experienced. In this safe relationship he can perceive for the first time the hostile meaning and purpose of certain aspects of his behaviour, and can understand why he has felt guilty about it and why it has been necessary to deny to awareness the meaning of this behaviour" (p. 41).

In contrast to Freud, Dr. Anthony Storr, in his book Art of Psychotherapy (1979) writes: "Since the therapist forms part of a reciprocal relationship, albeit of a specialised kind, he cannot maintain the kind of detachment which characterises the scientist conducting a scientific experiment. Understanding other people is, inescapably, a different enterprise from understanding things; and those who attempt to maintian towards people the kind of detached attitude which they might adopt towards things render themselves incapable of understanding others at all."

Instructions to peddle warmth somehow smack suspiciously of the salesman and the do-gooder. The recipient is apt to be left feeling "Why the hell am I the only person in the world to be feeling mean, angry, envious and ungrateful?" Treating people as people is another matter. Anyone needing to stress the importance of a warm, positive regard must have known the inclination towards cold, negative feelings to throw the former into perspective.

Each therapist must develop his own type of encounter with his patients. I find that my own approach varies subtly with each individual patient. There are some who feel the danger of suffocation faced with too much warmth. They need to feel that they are kept safely at a certain, consistent distance so that they cannot overpower the therapist or be overpowered by him. Others are so excitable in their transference love that they do not need the slightest encouragement in warmth, and in fact only need to get a little of it to unleash their feelings in physical action rather than make any attempt to understand and examine them through verbalisation.

With monosyllabic borderline schizophrenics I find it often necessary for me to relinquish the passive role and to offer them a model of a fully expressive, responsive fellow human being. Then after a time they may accept the model and begin to open up and express themselves more freely and spontaneously, whereupon the therapist can settle down to a quieter, more containing role. However, he must keep a careful eye open as to whether this stance is really freeing the patient or whether it is making her withdraw further in envy.

Bion (1977) describes the therapist as being a "container" and the patient as being "contained." If the patient can feel that her feelings can be accepted and held in this way, then she can later experience and contain them herself and therein not need to block them off and turn them into symptoms or causes of bizarre or anti-social behaviour.

Being a container is not synonymous with being a lavatory into which feelings are going to be evacuated and flushed away never to be seen or felt again. The therapist will contain and transmute the emotion making it able to be taken back and reflected on by the patient. For example: a manic-depressive patient said that she had felt fine when she left her home, but as she approached the therapist's flat she was overcome with a depressive mood. Although she did not want to explore this in the session, she did begin to cry and let it all out, saying that she felt as if she was depositing her depression with the therapist, whereupon she informed the therapist that she wanted to terminate the therapy. She then rushed out in the middle of the session as if she had flushed her depression down the therapist's "lavatory." The therapist subsequently wrote to the patient explaining the situation, and the patient replied that she felt that she was in need of help with these turbulent feelings, realising now that it had not been possible to dispose of her depression in this way.

If the therapist feels frankly cold and hating towards one of his more impossible patients, he needs to be able to contain these feelings and try and understand them while he continues to work devotedly with the patient. Occasionally he may find that the patient loads him with more negative emotion than he can take alone, in which case he may want to work through some of this emotion with a colleague or a psychotherapist.

Personally, though I have worked with patients who evoked in me strong feelings of revulsion and even hate, I do not think that I could work with a patient who I did not also find lovable in some way. In this work I feel at first that I am searching for some kind of treasure. I am seeking for some little clue as to how this patient's true self could develop; the clue may be in a musical phrase or a facial expression or a pregnant sentence. Before I have recognised this clue it is as if I am working on a two dimensional plane. When the intimation of her potential is revealed, suddenly the picture is different and we seem to be working in three dimensions. That clue belongs to the future and to the past, and is somehow the link between the two.

While being aware of the need to allow oneself to be warm and to be a human being, it is important to stress that it is the patient's inner world that the therapist should be exploring. The therapist should be aware of his own feelings and inner life but these will not be the subject of their explorations.

In Volume 12 of the Complete Works, Freud wrote: "The doctor should be opaque to his patients, and, like a mirror, should show them nothing but what is shown to him" (p. 118). The idea of this opacity is that this makes it easier for the patient to project her feelings on to the therapist and for these then to be worked out between them as they represent the patient's unfinished business from past relationships.

The patient may try to turn the investigation round the other way and explore the therapist's inner life and circumstances, but she will be repeatedly turned gently and firmly back to the investigation of her own inner and outer life. If she finds that she cannot intrude into private areas of the therapist's life then she will also discover that she too has the freedom to choose whether other people will be allowed to intrude into her inner and outer life. This will give her greater strength and independence.

Thus, although the therapist may be friendly and well-disposed towards his patient, he is not a friend---nor is he a teacher, a marriage partner, a judge, a lover, or a lavatory. He is not there to advise, or criticise, or applaud, though he may from time to time do a bit of each judiciously. He is a therapist who will work towards making the patient whole through their mutual exploration of her inner life with more understanding and clarification, his receptivity in words and attitude and reciprocity in music.

No discussion of the therapist-patient relationship would be complete without a clarification of the four levels of meeting: the working alliance, the transference, the musical relationship and the role-free human relationship. Greenson (1967) describes the working alliance as "the relatively non-neurotic rational relationship between patient and analyst which makes it possible for the patient to work purposefully in the analytic situation."

With the hospitalised patient, some of the function of the working alliance is taken over by the hospital staff who remind the patient to attend her session on time, look after her in between sessions and pay the therapist for his services. Certain kinds of patient form poor working alliances and can be difficult to work with on a private basis. For example the manic-depressive patient described earlier, who walked out in the middle of her session. In such cases, there is the danger of the split between the manic part of the patient wanting to act in a way that would not benefit the depressive part.

Greenson, in the same work, describes the transference as "the experiencing of feelings, drives, attitudes, fastasies and defences toward a person in the present which do not befit that person but are a repetition of reactions originating in regard to significant persons of early childhood, unconsciously displaced on to figures in the present. The two outstanding characteristics of a transference reaction are: it is a repetition and it is inappropriate." In fact it is a distortion.

The therapist, being in the parent position, will draw strong transference feelings on to himself, and will need to be aware of them. He can either work with the transference, helping the patient to understand towards whom these feelings belong in the past, or he can be aware that there are these feelings but not try to resolve them or point them out to the patient, in which case he is offering a transference cure. Many doctors operate on this basis. As an example of the former method of working, a young wife with conversion hysteria came to analytical music therapy fortnightly and said how jealous she was of her husband's new, blond, female business partner. The therapist brought this into the transference by saying she thought this patient was jealous of the patient who came in her alternate weeks off and then linked this with feelings about her younger brother. They played some music about the business partner which brought out hate, anger and resentment.

Sometimes the transference is loving and is called positive

transference, but sometimes it is negative, in which case it is particularly necessary to work with it or the patient may opt out of therapy before the important work is done. Very often positive tranference will mask its negative counterpart, and it is only when the patient has become confusingly aware of both that the work really goes forward. Negative transference can also mask the positive. Sometimes the feelings will be split between the beloved therapist and a detested outside figure. But these negative feelings must also be brought into the therapeutic relationship so that they can be worked with and understood. Sometimes the opposite happens and an outside figure is idealised. Freud wrote: "The psycho-analyst knows that he is working with explosive forces and that he needs to proceed with as much caution and conscientiousness as a chemist" (Complete Works, Volume 12, p. 170).

However, not all feelings that a patient has towards her therapist have the distortion of transference; and transference feelings are not exclusively experienced by patients in therapy. Most people carry over emotional attitudes towards their parents, to their beloveds. Many unequal relationships such as lawyer/client, conductor/violinist, priest/parishioner and so on carry traces of parent/child relationships.

Therapists have reactions too, and these are often referred to as a countertransference. Countertransference can be defined as all of the unconscious reactions that a therapist has towards a patient, and especially to the patient's transference. Much more will be said about this in another essay.

The musical level of relationship is reciprocal. Feelings are exchanged musically and the therapist will often be quite frank about his countertransference reactions via the music. At this level the therapeutic couple are closest together at the most unconscious depth. For example patients with a deep fear of closeness may play in such a way that it is impossible for the therapist to play with them. Their unconscious subtle arhythmic variations throw the therapist off, however hard he tries to be with them. If one considers that the therapist is skilled in accompanying and quartet-playing this is a remarkable feat on the part of the patient.

Skynner (1976) says: "The prime necessity is for the therapist to receive the projection without being taken over by it and acting it out, so that he can maintain his own identity and respond in a way that is related to the expectations inherent in the model projected, but which is different and, hopefully, (if the therapist is more mature or healthy than the person on whom the original model was based), a more accurate and effective guide to dealing with the world" (p. 79).

The therapist must be strong and stable enough to maintain his own identity but remain vulnerable to the message of these projections. The negative transference will often at first only show itself in the music. For example, a 40 year old woman with recurrent depression was at first very timid and submissive in the verbal part of the therapy but took a sadistic delight in playing pianissimo on the most delicate instruments and then suddenly whacking the big tom-tom and watching me jump. Later this aggression came into her words.

It is through the white heat of the positive transference that the patient is able to take on emotional tasks that she formerly shirked. Through this she gains the courage to re-make her life and re-forge her destiny. Her struggle will always be in the direction of the possession of the loved object (in this case the therapist) but through the rigorous lack of gratification this aim will be deflected on to work with the problems of external life and to finding more satisfying physically-reciprocal relationships. Freud wrote: "This struggle between the doctor and the patient, between the intellect and instinctual life, between understanding and seeking to act is played out almost exclusively in the phenomena of the transference" (Complete Works, Volume 12, p. 108).

When the role-free human relationship is experienced, with the least possible distortion, the patient is ready to leave.

Essay Eight

Transference and Countertransference

The Nature of Transference

In his early work, Freud referred to the phenomenon of trans-ference as "wrong association," as he recognised that some of his patients were regarding him with emotions that were relevant to previous relationships in their lives, usually parental. At first this transference, as he soon called it, was regarded as an embarrassment and hindrance in the work of remembering forgotten traumas. From 1917 Freud came to the full realisation that transference presented the patient with a golden opportunity to relive the past in a way that would be educative, giving her insight into habitual emotional reactions and the possibility of growth and change within the now therapeutic relationship. He wrote in "Analytic Therapy" (1917) that the trans-ference becomes a kind of battleground between the libido and all the forces opposing its expression, and that the relationship with the analyst was the meeting place for this struggle.

Within the transference the patient repeats emotional behaviour which she used in the past as a defence against remembering the pain and anxiety of her earlier life. The therapist, however, does not react in the way that the early object---whether parent or parent substitute---did in her early life, and his response and interpretations enable the patient to liberate herself from her repetition compulsion and begin to experiment with new ways of acting and responding. The insight that the patient gains helps her through the stages of: a) understanding how and why she acted as she did emotionally in the past; b) how she is acting in the present (without being able to change); and c) how she is about to act, but now with the possibility of changing her behaviour, and ultimately relieving herself of the necessity of acting in this way in the present in place of remembering the past.

The power of the emotions evoked in the positive transference urges the patient forward to struggle with the tasks of life where she may hope to find the gratification that is not provided to her within the therapeutic relationship. It also gives her the courage to face the painful emotions which she had repressed.

,   Negative transference, doubting or disliking the therapist, or sexual tranference, desiring him sexually, was seen by Freud as a form of resistance, or defence, as one would express it today.

Certainly it is essential for the therapist to uncover negative transference, work with it in the sessions and discover from whence it originates. If he does not manage to do this, the patient may act out against all kinds of innocent authority and nurturing figures and get herself into serious trouble or negative emotional involvement. Furthermore, there is the risk that she will break off the therapy at the very point when she most needs to continue it. Similarly, the sexual transference should be uncovered and reflected on or there will be the probability of the patient acting out these desires compulsively in numerous ill-advised and hasty sexual encounters.

Of course the behaviour of the therapist is very important in evoking certain kinds of transference. Reassuring motherly behaviour, including the giving of advice, engenders regressive behaviour in the patient. Siding with her defences ensures getting nowhere comfortably. Cold, supercilious behaviour may evoke a negative transference or the sudden departure of the patient; on the other hand an overwarm approach may frighten some patients too, and engender a negative mother transference. All therapists have their own styles depending on their individual personalitites; but it is always useful for a therapist to be aware of his or her main tendency and work to counteract this when necessary.

As the patient is projecting her internal objects on to the therapist, it follows that when their relationship is allowed to change, her relationship to her re-introjected internal objects will have altered and she should eventually be able to live much more comfortably with herself and with others.

Many, but not all, psychotherapists work on the premise that all that the patient speaks about refers to her relationship to the therapist and her nearest objects. All her related external events are also interpreted in this way and such interpretations are termed "transference interpretations." This approach helps to focus the patient's emotion firmly in the therapeutic relationship where it is worked out between them. (It can feel extremely claustrophobic and frustrating to the patient. For example if the patient has left her vest off and is feeling too cold and when asking to have the fire on is told that what she is saying is that she would like their relationship to be somewhat warmer, it can feel to some patients like an invitation to experience a psychotic denial of her physical awareness).

It is open to music therapists who have had experience of this kind of therapy to use transference interpretations in the verbal part of the therapy, but whether they do or not, the improvised duets offer special opportunities for the expression and exploration of transference emotions.

With the use of imagination exercises using improvised music, the music therapist has a useful tool with which to uncover the origins and the full emotional colouring of the negative or positive transference. The patient can improvise in the role of the therapist, while the therapist plays the patient; in this way the patient may find herself regaining her projection and being in touch with the real owner of these emotions. She can, if she is free enough, fantasise about what she would like to do with or to the therapist, and notice what ego she feels herself to be during this exercise.

As these feelings and fantasies are allowed to develop, the patient's capacity for loving grows and the therapist's tolerance and warmth help her to judge herself more favourably and to dare to reach out to others and begin to love nonjudgmentally in turn.

When I was a music therapy student an astonishing doctor and lecturer said: "Transference? I certainly do not allow anything like that to take place." But transference is always there, not only between patients and therapists but it can be observed in people's relationships with their priests, hairdressers, head waiters, chiropodists and teachers to name but a few in the nurturing or parental role. One cannot avoid it and, indeed, the therapist ignores it at his peril, though when he is aware of it, he has the right to decide in what way to use it. For example, he would probably choose not to make any transference interpretations if he were taking a patient for therapeutic tuition, although he might be aware that his patient was viewing him as her strict father and he would be making a point of mitigating this role and/or interpreting it.

To receive a patient's love with humility, knowing that one has it in trust for her loving relationships of the future, and to receive her hate with compassion, knowing that it was her badly-bruised love in the past which was longing to be healed and offered to life again, are important aspects of working with the transference.

If these attitudes are not maintained, the therapist can either feel unrealistically elated at being the recipient of so much adulation, or, sensing that this love is not for him, treat the patient's feelings with withering contempt.   Similarly he can feel hate in retaliation to the patient's hate.   But here we are entering the realm of the counter-transference.

Racker (1968) describes three distinct forms of countertransfer-ence.   The first is the therapist's own transference distortions in his relationship to the patient.   The second, which he calls "complementary identification" is caused by the therapist identifying with the patient's internal objects which she has projected on to him.   The third, which he calls "concordant identification" are "those psychological contents that arise in the analyst by reason of the empathy achieved with the patient and that really reflect and reproduce the latter's psychological contents."   Incidentally, the first paper written about the usefulness of countertransference as a psychoanalytic "tool" was by Paula Heimann in 1950.

For purposes of simplicity I shall call these "tools" counter-transference, c-countertransference and e-transference (Priestley 1985a) and will devote a separate section to each.   Because, generally speaking, in analytic literature only one word is used for all three phenomemon, a certain amount of confusion has arisen.   They actually feel different in the therapist when they occur and need to be clarified for the newly qualified therapist.   Winnicott (1965) wrote, "Would it not be better at this point to let the term countertransference revert to its meaning of that which we hope to eliminate by selection and analysis and the training of analysts?   This would leave us free to discuss the many interesting things that analysts can do with psychotic patients who are temporarily regressed and dependent, for which we could use Margaret Little's term: 'The analyst's total response to the patient's needs'."   But personally I prefer to use one simple word, the e-countertransference, in place of this eight-word phrase, besides, the use of e-countertransference is not soley the prerogative of analysts.

Countertransference

There are only four references to countertransference in the complete works of Freud as compared to seventy-seven references to transference (excluding in the notes). It is not clear from these references whether he distinguished between different kinds of countertransference, but it seems likely that he was talking about countertransference and e-countertransference when, in 1910, he wrote that analysts had become aware of countertransference and that it should be recognised and overcome during analysis.

Later, in "Observations on Transference Love" (Complete Works, Volume XII, 1915) speaking of the temptations involved in working with enamoured female patients, he wrote that in his opinion the analyst should not give up the neutrality towards the patient which had been acquired by keeping the countertransference in check.

Both the idea of "overcoming" and "keeping the transference in check" contain within them the essential ingredient of awareness of the distortion, for which purpose Freud advocated personal analysis. More recently the help of a supervisor to point out the therapist's blind spots in his initial stages of professional work has been found to be of invaluable assistance. It seems unlikely here that Freud was thinking of e-countertransference because the therapist would not so much want to "overcome" and "keep in check" these concordant identifications as to understand them and make use of them in his interpretations.

Perhaps the sparseness of early literature about classical countertransference was due to this feeling that it was something to overcome and check. Winnicott's terse remark on hate in the countertransference (1951) implies that it was an indication that the analyst needed more analysis. He said: "Well analysed therapists do not experience countertransference feelings of this nature." If so, this makes it extremely difficult for those therapists who do experience them to feel that they can go to someone more experienced in their field and ask for help. For the music therapist who has had an analysis, some analytical psychotherapy or possibly lengthy analytical music therapy, there is the possibility of self-analysis or, better still, working the situation through with the splitting technique with a colleague who has had some kind of training in this type of work. But for the music therapist who has had no such preparation there is the danger that the countertransference manifestation will not be recognised as something that needs to be understood and counteracted or simply not recognised at all, and the patient may suffer in the process.

Racker (1968) writes that positive transference usually evokes positive countertransference often with some manic feelings in the therapist, and again, by talion law, negative transference evokes negative countertransference often with some depressive feelings. However, one therapist known to me experienced feelings of deep contempt for his adoring patient and this was a manic defence against his sadness at not receiving the love that he yearned for from another source.

It seems fairly obvious that a negative countertransference should be analysed; as a therapist's opinion of himself as a therapist, or even as a human being, is lowered by active feelings of hate towards someone who is supposed to be in his care for the purpose of healing. But it is less obvious that his positive countertransference should also be examanined as it might fall into seductive patterns of an early symbiotic relationsip, making growth and the development of a healthy sense of separateness difficult or impossible for his patient to achieve.

Envy can be a difficult emotion to battle with in the counter-transference. The patient may be significantly better off financially than the therapist who, coming back from a modest holiday in the country, may find his feelings difficult to contain in the face of his patient's descriptions of her neurotic misery in the Caribbean. If he is single and sometimes lonely, his patient's tales of her trials with her widespread and loving family may be hard to bear. The patient may be better endowed by nature with more beauty, stronger physique and greater talents in the arts. The therapist will have to examine the roots of his envy and see what past pain is feeding it.

A special complication can be caused by a triangle situation with the patient and another person involved in the same case, often a doctor or a psychologist. It would not be unusual if there is sparse feedback from the medical colleague, and the therapist's unconscious can view the patient and doctor as an excluding parental couple and feel demeaned and castrated. Consequently he may find it difficult to work with the patient, experiencing his authority as a therapist as being undermined. Alternatively, his unconscious can view the couple as being his mother and a younger sibling getting together in some mutually gratifying situation behind his back, and leaving him with therapeutically destructive jealousy feelings in the session.

People take up therapy for various unconscious reasons. Often there is a feeling of having damaged an object (loved person) in the past, frequently in a destructive unconscious phantasy which may have collided unfortunately with a reality such as death, illness or prolonged absence. Thus the therapy is an act of reparation to the object, and an affirmation of the self as a healing person. Therefore, faced with the patient who refuses to progress, all the therapist's old feelings of destructiveness, and the guilt they produce, can well up into an emotion of hate towards the patient. The patient's refusal to improve becomes a hideous proof not just of the therapist's inability to heal, but of his total unfitness for the healing profession. He hates himself and the patient with him. In some hospital wards dying patients are viewed in this way and in consequence experience emotional isolation though they may be physically well cared for. Dying is felt as a failure for the medical team. It is the unforgivable response to therapy. Perhaps that is why people say there is such a good atmosphere in some hospices where living fruitfully till death is the accepted programme. With other therapists, themselves childless, therapy is seen as proof of their ability to triumph over their own parent in being a perfect mother. They have problems about separation, and for their patients the unforgivable response is to recover and leave the therapist. They become locked in the perfect-mother-to-perfect-child symbiosis which, though healing and even necessary for a time, can become stagnating, stultifying and ultimately mutually destructive

Racker (1968) describes the masochistic therapist who puts all his sadism into his patient and then lets the patient control him to the point of being unable to charge her a reasonable fee, terminate sessions on time or make a useful amount of interjections. In fact the therapist opts out of good parenthood. When the therapist can explore further his own aggressive feelings and feel able to make use of them creatively in the sessions, the therapy can improve remarkably.

The music therapist will probably first be aware of countertransference as an intimation that the emotions in the therapeutic dyad are becoming unmanageable. He finds himself in the grip of feelings that he cannot understand and yet he feels controlled by them. He cannot get the case out of his mind, it intrudes into his free time and the twilight hours. He may feel that he has to justify himself and his handling of the case and finds that he is having inner arguments with himself about it at odd private moments.

It is then necessary to examine the case and see whether there is anything in it that could suggest that his unconscious is seeing this patient as a figure from his past. The unconscious sees only infinite sets. Thus the therapist's arrogant older man patient may become confused with an invidious uncle who has chastised him as a child, together with all the other arrogant older men in his imagination. It takes patient, conscious thought and discrimination, or what Blanco calls asymmetrical thinking, to disentangle them and see his patient only as his unique, original self. It is in this process of disentanglement that some analytical music therapy with a more experienced therapist comes into its own. By improvising in the role of his patient, the therapist may come to discover who, from the past, he has come to confuse with this patient. In fact he retrieves his projection.

Then, doing some splitting exercises alternately in the role of the patient and himself, together with his senior colleague in the opposite roles, he may again begin to get in touch with the residue of emotion from his original relationship and work honestly on this. It may take him a very short time to gain insight into the current situation, and the therapist may feel that this is all that he needs. Digging deeper into the layers of unexpressed emotion with its residue of resentment and pain may, however, be a longer business; but always uniquely valuable to his work in the long run.

In this way every patient can teach his therapist something about himself, especially those who he finds most difficult. In the hardest cases, it is the painful growth by both therapist and patient that achieves the therapeutic results as countertransference always points to valuable areas for self-development. The therapist who ignores it cheats both himself and his patient.

Complementary Identifications
or C-Countertransferences

Complementary identifications, or c-countertransferences, occur when the therapist identifies with one of the patient's introjects; or, as one might say, when he introjects his patient's introject and is taken over by it. For example: he might behave like his patient's spoiling mother or strict father. It is, of course, an unconscious process, but how does it make itself known to the therapist? In some cases, he is not consciously aware of it and the unfortunate patient is subjected not to a "corrective emotional experience" but a negative affirmatory experience as the therapist and patient re-enact an unfortunate relationship from the patient's past. (Note that in c-countertransference the situation is a repetition of the patient's past, not that of the therapist's as in Freudian countertransference).

The c-countertransference may come to the therapist's awareness through an uneasy question of "Why am I doing/saying this?" and a vague feeling of acting out of character, not once, but over and over again with this one particular patient. To a certain extent most therapists change subtly with each patient and this is part of their normal sensitivity; but in the case of c-counter-transference, they may be aware of somehow being pushed into a change that they do not like. Of course when it is a harsh or cold or aggressive way of acting, a warm therapist might be quickler to discover something was wrong; but he can also be taken over by an adoring, spoiling or overprotective introject which might be a little more difficult for such a therapist to disentangle.

Some of the early analysts purposely allowed themselves to act out some of the c-countertransferences in order to speed the development of a strong transference. For example: with a patient who had had a strict father such an analyst would start by being extremely strict and gradually become milder to the point where the patient could dare to interact with him and learn to stand up to her external or introjected father figure. However, this artificial manoevre was not generally approved of or considered necessary.

Where c-countertransference is suspected, the music therapist can find it helpful to ask the patient to make a musical sculpture of her

family of origin.   She will place various instruments to represent
different members of her family, at distances from her seat that
represent how near or far she feels emotionally to each one.   The
therapist then sits in the patient's seat at the xylophone and the patient
goes round to each instrument in turn improvising music to describe
how she feels that each relative feels or felt about her.   When she
comes to the one whose introject the therapist is identifying with, he
may sense that this is the character that he is being forced to imitate;
and it can be possible for them to have a fruitful discussion about this
character's influence on her life, both in the past and in the present
through the medium of the introject and externally.   Although this may
not free the therapist entirely of his identification, he will at least be
more aware of what is going on; and sometimes the patient may also
even be able to point out how she is experiencing his behaviour as
being like her original object.   This can bring about insight and
changes on both sides.

Racker (1968) explains that the complementary identifications
come about by the patient treating the analyst (or therapist) as her
internal or projected object and him feeling treated as this object and
behaving in identification with it.   He explains that there seems to be
a relationship to the concordant (or e-countertransference) here in that
the less he is aware of this the more likely he is to be taken over by
the complementary identifications (or c-countertransference).

Through the resolution of the c-countertransference the
therapist may become increasingly open to the more empathic e-
countertransference and much can be worked through and learnt by the
patient during this process once the couple's insight is developed.   It
is possible in this way for a patient to develop a more constructive and
less self-destructive relationship to the introject of a relative long since
dead but still a powerful negative influence internally.

After the therapist has realised the relationship of the patient to
this introject, he can gradually learn to accept the patient's projection
consciously, but change its character subtly so that the patient learns
to relate to it (through him) in a more fruitful way, first externally and
then internally when she re-introjects it.   However, even with insight,
it can be extremely difficult for the therapist to shed the c-countertransference.   Nevertheless, once realised and struggled with, the

c-countertransference offers a rich field for the development of the patient's ability to relate to others and to live with herself more peacefully. Unrealised, it leads to a mutually destructive situation for the therapeutic couple. There is, with c-countertransference, the feeling of the therapist being diminished, of a dwindling of his powers of freedom, insight and emotional breadth. Of course, every therapist will experience c-countertransference differently; but it is useful for a therapist to clarify the experience in his own mind in some way, so as to be able to recognise it more easily when it occurs again.

Privately I imagine this condition to be similar to existing in a soft-shelled egg to which pressure is being applied that forces a certain behaviour out of me toward the unfortunate patient. Dr. J. W. Redfearn (1992) says that c-countertransference feels only too natural to him; the patient evokes it and accommodates herself to it from years of habit. However, the feeling of pressure and enclosure are very real to me though I realise that this image is purely personal. But awareness is at the core of all forms of countertransference, and if creating an image helps the therapist to focus it then he should not hesitate to do so. Clothed in such hygienic analytic terms, these experiences sound quite pat and manageable---in reality they can be extremely spooky to the uninitiated therapist experiencing them for the first time.

E-Countertransference

Racker (1968) writes about concordant identification (e-countertransference) as "the resonance of the exterior to the interior" (p. 128). This delighted me, as e-countertransference has always given me the image of a plucked string instrument (the patient) whose music resonates on its sympathetic strings (the therapist), and the very word concordant, which literally means "with string," affirms this image. The therapist may find that either gradually as he works, or with a suddeness that may alarm him, he becomes aware of the sympathetic resonance of some of the patient's feelings through his own emotional and/or somatic awareness. Often these are repressed emotions that are not yet available to the patient's conscious awareness but they can also be feelings which are in the process of becoming conscious, in which case they may be very dynamic and fluent in the therapist, especially when he is improvising.

Working, as music therapists do, with the emotions of the patient, it is generally to the emotions that the therapist develops this response. With physical healers there can be what the Russian healers call the "echo effect" during which the healer responds to the pain of the patient by feeling a corresponding discomfort in his own body. I have met several English spiritual healers who made use of this response, and I myself have also been aware of some of my patients' headaches when they first sat in the chair opposite me before they began to speak. The response often occurs in mirror-fashion, that is, the patient's left side being felt on the therapist's right side.

While not having done any research into this phenomenon, it does seem to be more widespread than one might imagine from the little that is spoken about it even in therapeutic circles. Possibly this is because it is difficult to explain and not available for testing because of its unreliability, for example Russian healers have said that thunderstorms put their mechanism out of action temporarily. There is also a form of it in the couvade, a primitive custom, where husbands take to their beds when their wives are in labour, and then experience the birth contractions as if he is giving birth, even to the point where the wife may have little awareness of serious discomfort herself.

In the case of the analytical music therapist, where the response is usually purely emotional, I have only a limited number of examples to draw on. When lecturing on e-countertransference the therapist invariably gets asked, "How do you know that they are the patient's feelings?". My own answer to that is because I usually experience these particular feelings in a very concentrated form in the region of the solar plexus in a manner that I do not experience my own emotions which are felt to be more diffuse. (In conversation with the late Dr. Louis Zinkin, a Jungian analyst, and Jean Hindson, a psychotherapist, they agreed that they felt the patient's emotions in the same area themselves while giving therapy.) Added to this is the therapist's awareness of his own emotions which he has learned about during the analytical work on himself, plus the intellectual computations as to whether these feelings could conceivably be the repressed or nearly surfacing emotions of the patient at that particular time.

Bion (1955) writes of the use of the e-countertransference with psychotic patients: "The analyst who essays, in our present state of ignorance, the treatment of such patients, must be prepared to discover that for a considerable proportion of analytic time the only evidence on which an interpretation can be based is that which is afforded by the countertransference." It is clear that he is referring to the e-countertransference.   Later he writes: "The objection that I project my conflicts and phantasies onto the patient cannot and should not be easily dismissed.   The deference must lie in the hard facts of the analytic situation, namely that in the present state of pychoanalytic knowledge the analyst cannot rely on a body of well-authenticated knowledge. Further, he must assume that his own analysis has gone far enough to make disastrous misinterpretations unlikely."

This reinforces the belief that the therapist can gain a great deal from some protected and concentrated work on his own emotions, and this will help in his assessment of the situation when he does find himself experiencing e-countertransference.   This phenomenon is not restricted to certain persons, but can easily develop without understanding or insight even in children who may respond to the experienced environmental emotions with bilious attacks, asthma or other psychosomatic disorders.

On the other hand some well-trained therapists may find these emotional echoes extremely hard to tune in to, and may have to make a special effort of self-examination to get any personal idea of which emotions their patients may be repressing at any given moment. Certain therapists find some emotions easier to respond to than others. One therapist found that with anger, panic, deep sadness or elation it was quite simple to separate the patient's emotion from his own quite neatly.   The emotion that he found really crippling was a hopeless feeling of inadequacy.   He said that he had a real battle with himself when working with patients who handed him this emotion.   But when he had succeeded in isolating it and handing it back to the patient (always in words as he had not yet found out how to express this particular emotion musically) he had always had important results, with the patient taking over the struggle and no longer using her energy only in projection.   This led to an immediate mitigation of the therapist's own feelings as he could understand that he was not only resonating but also identifying with this baffling emotion in himself.

The e-countertransference is a useful tool which is written about by several anaylsts. Rosenfeld (1955) wrote: "In my opinion the unconscious intuitive understanding by the psychoanalyst of what a patient is conveying to him is an essential factor in all analysis, and depends on the analyst's capacity to use his countertransference as a kind of sensitive 'receiving set'. In treating schizophrenics who have such great verbal difficulties, the unconscious intuitive understanding of the analyst through the countertransference* is even more important, for it helps him to determine what it is that really matters at that moment. But the analyst should also be able to formulate consciously what he has unconsciously recognised, and to convey it to the patient in a form that he can understand."

His asterisk refers to a quotation from Paula Heimann (1950) in which she hypothesizes "that the analyst's emotional response to his patient within the analytic situation represents one of the most important tools for his work. The analyst's countertransference is an instrument of research into the patient's unconscious."

The therapist's e-countertransference depends on his sensitivty and his freedom to experience the incoming emotions. But his ability to formulate it consciously and use it to the benefit of his patient depends on his clarity of thinking. If he becomes flooded by his patient's repressed emotion and unable to think and interpret in the face of it, he will be in a very bad way indeed, extremely uncomfortable, and with the therapy in a totally static state.

Nevertheless e-countertransference can be difficult to interpret, and the power of the emotional reactions do sometimes block clear thinking temporarily. It takes experience to learn to keep quite still, making no attempt to rid oneself of the discomfort these emotions may produce, and ask oneself what they may be meaning to the patient and how to hand them back in an acceptable form, be it musical or verbal.

Besides the inner awareness of the patient's emotion, some therapists experience a certain disturbance in various parts of their bodies. For example a sexual e-countertransference can be experienced as a kind of disturbing warmth in the genital region which is quite different from the normal sexual excitation on arousal. About this Racker (1968) writes: "In passing, I would like to mention that at times the analyst - if his unconscious is well-connected with that of the patient - may perceive her repressed or split-off sexual excitement through sexual sensations of his own, in a certain way 'induced' by the patient."

Certain very disturbed patients produce in the therapist feelings of acute discomfort in the head, which are strongest on initial contact and which disappear after weeks or a few months of weekly sessions. I cannot explain this but it seems to be a reaction to a disturbed function of some kind in the patient. Certain states of repressed anger or tears in the patient can produce feelings of tightness---almost choking---in the therapist's throat. This can be quite unpleasant for the therapist but is easily dispersed by expressing that emotion in music.

The degree of unusualness of the therapist's experience is related to the patient's degree of being split off from her emotion. Thus psychotherapists, who at present skim the cream of available patients, will probably feel their e-countertransference reactions to be more connected and natural. But even if a music therapist should be working with a more integrated and intelligent patient, he should beware of rationalising his emotions and ask himself, "Is the patient pushing this into me?". He must always be watching out for the various forms of countertransference.

Some e-countertransference manifestations however only appear while the music therapist is improvising. One response to a strong unconscious crippling feeling of inadequacy and panic can be a feeling of near-paralysis in the fingers of the therapist which can make playing extremely difficult. In this case the therapist can only free himself from this response by carefully bringing this feeling of paralysing impotence into the awareness of the patient verbally. It is sometimes easier to talk about the emotion in the e-countertransference if the therapist first expresses it in their improvisation and then draws the patient's attention to it saying something like: "There seemed to be a feeling of excitement (or sadness or anger) so I put it into the music." Then if the patient is ready to own it she will. If not, it does not matter, they can come back to it later on.

Another curious e-countertransference manifestation which can come only during an improvisation, is the e-countertransference tune.

This is different from the already composed tunes that one of my colleagues says come to her while improvising with patients and which she introduces into the music. Usually on examination one finds that the title or words of these tunes (usually songs) are relevant to the situation. The e-countertransference tune usually turns itself into one which the therapist plays with great conviction, and the patient usually listens with rapt attention and accompanies it very softly. One patient said, on hearing the playback, "When you played that, it was me." If the patient is not ready, however, she will not listen, and this is a lonely feeling for the therapist. Some of Beethoven's last themes have the quality of e-countertransference tunes perhaps representing the lost faith and hope of suffering humanity.

It takes years of experience in one-to-one therapy to develop this awareness of e-countertransference into a really useful tool for the exploration of the patient's unconscious. It involves both willingness to experience deep and often uncomfortable states of emotion and also to develop mind control in the face of these experiences. It is not something that one can decide to have nothing to do with. If it is there, it is there with a message which can be decoded. Refusal to look at this message may leave the therapist in acute discomfort and the therapy in a state of stagnation.

E-countertransference offers a unique possibility for self-development for the therapist in his work; it offers a challenge to be met with great concentration and courage and it can bring a rich reward in the increased ability to understand and help his patients.

Clinical Examples

Transference

I was working with a 32-year-old man who was rehabilitating following hospitalisation with schizophrenia. He was very keen on betting on horse races, and this activity formed part of his very close relationship with his mother. At work, he and one of his mates would dash out to the bookmaker and place their bets for afternoon races and then listen surreptitiously to the results on a tiny radio. His talk about the subject briefly awakened my interest and I even placed a small bet on one of his hot tips for the Derby, and won at unremarkable odds (possibly an example of c-countertransference)! Then I subsequently forgot all about it. At the next big race, possibly the Grand National, he came in all pink and expectant to ask how I had done. His look of disappointment and let-down was truly pitiful when he realised that I had been totally unaware of the race being on that day and that I was not his mother and this little area of mutual excitement between them was a dead area between us. His music describing the race was quite erotic.

My verbal interchange with this man was on a supportive basis and I was hardly interpreting at all, working largely with imagination exercises to help to connect his inner and outer worlds, and reality rehearsals to help him to face his next step in life. But the knowledge of his mother transference helped me to be an alternative nonpossessive, liberating type of mother.

Classical countertransference

Until I read Dr. Searles' "Collected Papers on Schizophrenia and Related Subjects" (1965) I thought that countertransference, in the classical Freudian sense, was something more or less eliminated by a thoroughgoing analysis and that its appearance indicated that more analysis was needed. In one way I would agree with this but it can also be the self-analysis of an already well-analysed therapist. After all, the very awareness that such a countertransference exists, indicates a certain level of insight and self-knowledge in the therapist. Having this amount of insight will surely spur him on to examine where this countertranference comes from, working through the feelings either on his own or, as is often the case with me, with the help of a colleague through music therapy, or with my supervisor. The fact that I had been reading Searles prior to this experience allowed me to open myself to it without panic or dismay.

The patient with whom I was working was a young woman of thirty-two, single, intelligent, musical, and verbally expressive. She was slim, of medium height and had bushy brown hair. Somehow working with her I had several times to question my impulse to behave more as a friend than a therapist. In fact I once briefly related to her an episode from my own life to realise keenly that I had stepped out of the therapist's role by the baffled look on her face, even though it was in fact quite relevant to the subject under exploration. Some sessions later while she was talking eagerly about something, I saw her head replaced by the head of my near-twin half-sister with that same bushy brown hair. It remained for a second then slid away like a child's transfer turning again into my patient's face with the more pointed nose and sharp chin. So it was a sister countertransference. I took the message from the unconscious gratefully and worked on it with my supervisor the next day. The feeling behind it was that I did not want to work with this patient but to play as I had done with my half-sister. This discovery at once restored our professional relationship and I could give a friendly but warning nod to any sisterly feelings that still passed through my mind.

C-Countertransference and E-Countertransference

The patient was a forty-six year old woman working as a medical secretary. She lived alone in a London flat but went down to Oxford each Friday to spend the weekend with her older sister and mother, returning home late on Sunday. This left her only four evenings a week in her own flat to fit in domestic chores, social life, a church group and her weekly session with me. Being rather shy, with such severe feelings of inadequacy that these had led to a suicidal attempt two years before she started work with me, it was the social life that suffered.

When she was quite young she had played the violin and, on the whole, in our improvisations, she rejected the percussion instruments, except for an occasional interlude on the xylophone, in favour of the melodica (a simple wind instrument). The ability to sustain a melody line on this instrument seemed to be important to her.

In our verbal exchange I felt I was being compelled to take her over and tell her what to do, why and when to do it. I fought against this, being quite shocked at myself for such untherapeutic inclinations; and then realised that I had identified with the introjected controlling mother figure. The mother was, actually, still alive and still behaving in a not very enabling way. After we had some talks about how her mother and sister always made her feel helpless and inadequate, my compulsion to take her over somewhat abated; but was nevertheless always there lurking, waiting to push me in that direction when I least expected it and I would check myself in the upbeat to the act thinking "What am I doing?" This c-countertransference only took place during the verbal part of our therapy.

During our improvisation her melodica playing gradually developed from anxious little pipings to fluent, soul-searching phrases with little rhythmical experiments in the form of an added quaver pattern or mordent as decoration. The e-countertransference that I experienced was a transporting sense of elation. At first I saw no way of bringing this to an outward manifestation when I improvised mainly diatonically, and we seemed to be stuck in the same stale little world with this intense, soaring feeling of elation bursting in my inner self. Later on I started using clusters of dissonances which seemed to me to describe something of an ecstacy born of pain; this to me gave a more honest picture of the gestalt and relieved the pressure of my inside feeling. The patient said that before the playback she was totally unaware of my music anyway. I did not press the awareness of it on her at all but let things take their course. Later I said that there seemed to be a feeling of excitement that was not attached to anything particular. She replied that she did have a strange feeling of excitement that morning walking to the underground, and she had this from time to time. In simple words I connected this with a reaching back to the pre-ambivalent symbiosis with the mother.

Later on we came to speak of her relationship with her father. She experienced him as always thinking she was "pretty useless" intellectually following a childhood illness, operations and missed schoolwork. However, she did manage to pass two out of six of her O level exams. Her father's comment "It could have been worse," though it seemed quite friendly and comforting to me, she experienced it as cutting and devastating. We improvised on this, she in the role of father and me as her. Her playing was no longer fluent and gently exploring but now blaring sforzando, and it gave me no trace of elation but desperate feelings of being blocked and denigrated and generally not allowed to be. We discussed this and it was exactly the feeling that she had had in this relationship. She also eagerly assured me that she loved her father very much and that there were lots of jokes and games in the family; but her sister was regarded as the "clever one" while she was the "stupid one." This particular e-countertransference was, I believe, very much what she passed on to others generally in social intercourse with her awkward stops and piercing stares. It also could have been part of the reason why this aspect of her life was so unrewarding.

Another E-countertransference

The patient, a student-nurse of 31 on an acute male psychiatric ward, played with very little expression and talked in a very quiet voice. In her third (fortnightly) session she opted to sit sideways, upright, on the reclining chair and asked if she could play the piano rather than the xylophone. When asked about this she said that she felt vulnerable in the chair and liked to feel in control of things. I said that this was perhaps why she chose to be a nurse where her role as controlling was clearly defined. She said that she was otherwise a very passive person, easily giving up any will of her own and falling in with the wishes of others. She was like this with her widowed mother. During this conversation I had experienced strong, unmistakable sexual e-countertransference. I opened up this subject. She had had some sexual experience, but only in one brief encounter had she had any pleasure from it; unfortunately she did not see that man again. At the moment she did not think about sex at all, it was what "the others" did.

We improvised some music as "The Sexualising Others." She was on the piano and afterwards when we heard it played back we agreed that it was hideously ugly music. She had actually been screwing up her face while playing; it was how she had usually felt while having sexual intercourse, she said. But dynamically it was the most vivid music that she had produced. We were on the track of the repressed sexual energy which had made itself known to me so usefully during our discussion.

We finished the session with an improvisation in which she was her "Asexual Self" (on the instruments) and I played the piano as "The Sexual Others," very romantically and passionately. This time she said that she could play along with my music without screwing up her face, and neither felt cut off and envious, or involved. Perhaps she was in the position of a happy child who has a comfortable unconscious awareness of the parental intercourse. When we were discussing the two improvisations that we had just played, all traces of a sexual e-countertransference had vanished. I was thus aware that she had been put in touch with her sexual feelings to some degree, and that the e-countertransference had guided me to this repressed energy.

Essay Nine

More on Empathic Countertransference

In this essay, the term countertransference is used in the sense of the therapist becoming aware of his physically experienced resonance to unconscious or preconscious emotions in the patient, and not in the sense of the transference distortions of his own feelings and projections on to the patient (which for example, may make him feel for her as he did for his younger sibling). It is extremely confusing that there is only one word for both phenomena in the literature.

Countertransference, in the first sense, is known among Siberian healers as the "echo effect," in that the pain of the patient can be echoed in the healer's own body. I myself have experienced this both as the patient, when a healer located the pain in my body before I had told her where it was; and several times as therapist when a patient has sat down in the chair opposite me and I have immediately felt the pain and pressure of her headache that she had not yet spoken about. (I almost never have headaches myself). As our patients are more usually suffering from emotional rather than physical pain, the emotional echo is the usual form this kind of countertransference takes.

I would like to distinguish this echoing form of countertransference by the name "empathic-countertransference," or to take in the idea of the physical echo effect too, the "e-counter-transference. It is this form of countertransference that I refer to throughout this chapter because it is with this phenomenon that the analytical music therapist works as he expresses these hidden emotions and gives them back to the patient through his music and, where he thinks the patient is ready for this, discusses them with her after their improvisation or playback.

I would say that e-countertransference is an essential tool for the analytical music therapist and would agree with Paula Heimann (1950) who pointed out that the analyst's emotional response to the patient is one of the most important tools, and that countertransference is an instrument of research into the patient's unconscious.

If e-countertransference is one of the most important tools for the analyst, it is that much more important for the analytical music therapist, because he can work with it in additional ways. For example, I had recently started work with a schizophrenic lady in her early sixties. She had been very much shielded from dwelling upon her life's vicissitudes by her psychically overprotective but physically helpful and supportive sisters. When she improvised with me on such subjects as "Motoring," "Cats," "Ghosts" and "Dull Moments," all of which had come up in our talks, I experienced feelings of acute sadness which I could locate in an area around my solar plexus.

After the second time that we improvised, I began to tell her that there were feelings of sadness. The first time she hastened to assure me that they were not hers and that she was feeling quite cheerful. She said: "You said that because you knew I had been ill". I said that all my patients had been ill but that with some I felt anger, some joy and some sorrow. However, by our tenth session she had accepted some of this sadness and allowed herself to contemplate what she thought of as her "wasted life," and we took her expression of "Feeling Old" as a theme for the next improvisation. I found the sadness pouring out into my music and the patient playing closely with me in an interesting quaver-crochet rhythm that was much more alive than her usual dull thumping four beats to a bar. This thumping had been music with a defensive quality, whereas the quaver-crochet rhythm was an acceptance of the sad feelings which she heard in my music and tried to stay with though she, herself, could not initiate the expression of this deep sadness. At the same time I no longer had the physical feeling of sadness inside my solar plexus area. The music had moved it from that painful inner area outward into verbal sharing.

Although the patient's music showed that she was able to share this with me in music and therefore at a deeper level, her split between emotion and thought made her deny awareness of it. The point of working through her sadness in the therapy was to counteract her manic stance of living beyond her means, and using overspending as her only expressive outlet to blot out depressive thoughts and experiences--rather like overeating in other people. This musical mirroring back of the e-countertransference feelings is one of the methods of dealing with them that is unique to music therapy. For a psychotherapist to start talking in a sad voice would hardly be the same and might sound like cruel mockery.

Sometimes e-countertransference is experienced psychosomatically and the therapist has the job of decoding his own somatic sensations to get at the emotion that is being passed on. I had this experience in my earlier days of practice. The sensations could be quite alarming for it took a minute or so to realise that this was an e-countertransference reaction and to decide whether the time was ripe for an interpretation, that is, whether to allow more time for the patient to reach into herself for an awareness of this emotion or whether to disperse it in oneself by feeding it back to her through the music.

Many therapists besides myself have been aware of a resonance of choking sensations which usually point to an excess of anger or sadness in the patient at a hidden level. I had one particular patient with rapid moodswings, suicidal depressions and an extremely traumatic early history which my supervising psychotherapist at the hospital said pointed to a very poor prognosis. (This was a challenge to me and, in fact she did well professionally and personally during the latter part of the six and half years in which I treated her, and is still doing well twelve years later). She would often produce this kind of e-countertransference in me. Sometimes I could lay the feelings before her verbally but at other times I had to clutch at personal survival. I really felt that I would choke unless I could disperse these emotions echoed from her. In connection with this when my holistic therapist first worked on the jaw and throat area, I was astonished to feel that I was momentarily taken over by a great Wolf or Dog subpersonality. A huge savage roar came out of me and my hands involuntarily clawed at the floor mattress on which we worked. No doubt there is some simple scientific explanation for this but I was immediately reminded of Hazrat Inayat Khan's (1960) explanation of "muwakkals," the elemental beings who live on unreleased charges of emotion. And so when asked by my therapist what I thought happened, I answered "You released a muwakkal!" And though momentarily stunned by the experience, I did not feel unduly perplexed. I suppose it could have been something to do with an unde-briefed attack on my face by a female greyhound deprived of her pups when I was about 10, leaving a block between turning such physical sensations caused by anger into thoughts and thus words.

To go back to my patient: we improvised strange music with wide dynamics and the emotions were dispersed at once into the music--hers or mine or both--and we were then often able to get in touch with her deeper fears. At such moments I wondered how psychotherapists could cope, battling with the containment and expression of such powerful feelings verbally, when these can be experienced so uncomfortably in the body. Eleven years after my long analysis when I embarked on the more body-based holistic therapy, this helped me to clear the energy blocks to the physical expression of some of my own deepest and earliest traumas. I doubt if I could have coped with these powerful physical and emotional expressive and releasing experiences had I not understood their roots through my earlier analysis and had such a good rapport with my therapists.

Another example of somatic countertransference was with a patient who was suffering from a repressed paralysing feeling of impotence, though outwardly confident and superior in manner. She produced in me the startling reaction of a physical sensation that I could not play. My fingers seemed semiparalysed. At first the impact of this phenomenon was so powerful that I was struggling only to complete our improvisation. (This was earlier on when I understood less about e-countertransference). At that session I did not realise what was happening and certainly failed to interpret her feelings of impotence. However, I thought through the experience and at the next session I was ready for it. The sensation returned in our improvisation, my fingers felt half numb but this time I acknowledged that she was passing me her impotence. In the session that ensued I was able to get her to look at this and take some of it back. I had a slight repeat of the phenomenon one more time and after that she had reclaimed enough of this feeling for me to be free from these troubling physical messages in our music.

Of course it would be possible for another therapist, less sensitive to e-countertransference, to deduce intellectually that the first mentioned patient had some sad, depressed feelings causing her manic stance and overspending. But the e- counter-transference takes the therapist right into the hidden emotion, and its peculiar quality can be expressed most compellingly through his music when the time is right for this. Patients and others often ask: "Why are you always looking for something negative? Why can't you accept me as I am and build on that?" But unfortunately it is not really satisfactory to build on such unstable foundations, partly because there is always the danger of the so-called "return of the repressed," in this case a depression caused by these sad feelings, partly because the ego loses a considerable amount of energy in keeping these feelings repressed, and lastly because the therapist will not be the only person to be affected by the e-counter-transference. The patient may lose friends and even jobs when they notice that they get depressed when they see her and gradually drift away to protect themselves without quite knowing why they do this.

Earlier on, in the first four or five years of my work as a therapist, I sometimes had somatic e-countertransference experiences when working on wards of psychotic patients. While I sat enjoying my colleague's piano music or a patient's song, the unconscious mood of the ward seemed to permeate my feelings through my fingers and it was often extremely hard to govern them when I started to play my violin. If I played immediately on entering a ward, the physical response was minimal and even later on if I could use some good, strong marcato bowing I was able to cut through the woolly, weak or sometimes ungovernable effect on my fingers and play tolerably well. Thus I could start successfully by playing Kreisler's Preludium and Allegro but might have difficulty in beginning with Faure's Lullaby however much it might suit the atmosphere of the ward. During the last twelve years or so working in the psychiatric hospital I became more aware of the prevailing underlying atmosphere of fear or anger or despair in the disturbed restricted wards and my fingers were then relatively free of somatic e-countertransference. This was possibly a more developed and more normal state of awareness.

A feeling of inferiority has not otherwise transmitted itself to me from the patient in this somatic way but more often directly through my emotions. For example: I had a healthy, normal business man who came to see me for musical coaching and lessons on the rudiments of music. He had strong unconscious feelings of inferiority although he was externally confident, extroverted, and had an overcompensating personality. Every time I played the piano I was overwhelmed with these feelings of inadequacy. This was, in all fairness, rather confusing because I am not a very accomplished pianist. Though I have developed my own pianistic method in improvisation and was complimented on it most heartily by a German pianist, the violin was my first study, and it was at first hard to sort out my own realistic feelings of inadequacy from those that he was passing to me through the unconscious.

In 1914, Freud wrote that "it is a very remarkable thing that the unconscious of one human being can react upon that of another, without passing through the conscious" (1959, Volume 14, p. 194). The experience with this business man was earlier in my career when I knew less about e-countertransference. However, one evening I said to myself, "I'm no worse of a pianist than I ever was, I've passed my exams, I'm a good musician, this load of inadequacy doesn't belong to me, I'm not accepting it." I played with great emotion and power, almost physically thrusting these feelings of inadequacy from me. It had a remarkable effect on my client who sang superbly but afterwards was able to claim some of the feelings of inadequacy as his own.

Music is an admirable vehicle for conveying this kind of unconscious communication and making it possible for some of the therapy to be carried on at that level. In fact I believe that the business man was enabled to resolve enough of these feelings of inadequacy to be able eventually to win the hand of the lady of his choice and move away, thus terminating our musical relationship satisfactorily.

I am sometimes asked how a therapist knows that e-countertransference feelings are anything to do with the patient and not just his own emotions. Racker (1968) found that having an exaggerated confidence in what one's own unconscious is saying is less dangerous than repressing them or denying their value altogether. The longer I work at analytical music therapy, the more precise an instrument does the e-countertransference become. The dramatic somatic feelings in the fingers or the throat or the eroticized sensations in other parts of the body have a compelling quality that leads the therapist urgently to the source of the emotion. When one gets to know them, the emotional e-countertransference feelings have a totally different quality from one's own. These emotional, physical sensations can be very sharp and clear but localised in the area of the solar plexus or they can have a kind of misty, overhanging quality about them which is somewhat harder to recognise. They can also, especially with new patients, be sensed as patterns of discomfort in certain areas of the head. The worst head feelings I have experienced came when I was first in touch with a man severely afflicted with obsessional neurosis. These feelings did not even wait until he came into therapy but, as he sat by me discussing his wish for music therapy in the club where I had been speaking, I became aware of intensely distressed areas in my head. These sensations continued during the discussion section of the next eight to ten sessions of our work, always being dispersed by the music. After that I was no longer aware of them. Such sensations offer no clue as to what unconscious emotion may be needing to be examined and accepted but I nevertheless count them as e-countertransferences.

Other therapists have also admitted to experiencing these sensations with certain patients. The fact that such e-counter-transference reactions are apparently nameless in therapeutic circles--I was in no way prepared for them in my training--seems to indicate that we have here entered a taboo area bordering on the psychic which is unpredictable and therefore has not yet been considered a suitable subject for scientific research or delineation.

Without having experienced some analytic psychotherapy and having learnt to know oneself at a deep level, it might be very much more difficult to help the patient to reach her hidden emotion. Naturally e-countertransference can be experienced by anyone in any interpersonal situation, it is not the prerogative of therapists. It is sometimes used instinctively with great sensitivity by members of other caring professions. Certainly it is used very skillfully by some fortune tellers and Customs Officers who are quite psychodynamically innocent. But as Paula Heimann wrote (1968) "When the analyst in his own analysis has worked through his infantile conflicts and anxieties (paranoid or depressive) so that he can easily establish contact with his own unconscious, he will not impute to the patient what belongs to himself" (p. 81).

The therapist has to learn to carry the different unrealised aspects of the patient and with the added tool of music this is made somewhat less painful. It is almost as if music constitutes a helpful third party in the therapeutic relationship, bearing some of the intolerable burden of the emotion and making some of it easier to accept by sublimation into a musical creation. The music seems to say, "Listen, these emotions can be expressed and shared and contained. They can even be played with". And this is how we all began to learn to live. The words of Dr. Winnicott (1971) seem relevant here: "We find either that individuals live creatively and feel that life is worth living or else that they cannot live creatively and are doubtful about the value of living."

Though transference was discussed in some detail in Music Therapy in Action (Priestley, 1975), what was not discussed and I will mention here, is the subject of transference interpretations. Ordinary interpretations are, of course, making the unconscious conscious for the patient, but this particular kind of intervention by the therapist interprets everything that the client says about happenings or emotion between her and outside agents as being statements about her feelings about the relationship within the therapy. For example, if the patient were to ask to have the window open the analyst could interpret that she is feeling that what is happening in the therapy is too hot for her. Thus an emotion is immediately given an outlet within the present relationship and the client is given an opportunity to express her feelings in a direct rather than an oblique way. For some clients these interventions are an acceptable, vital and mutative form of emotional hot-housing. Others find them frustrating, enraging and reality-fleeing.

Unless an analytical music therapist has had an analyst (probably Kleinian) who interprets in this way, he will find this style of work well-nigh impossible to carry out. In any case, transference interpretations can be difficult to think out and present in words, and unless they come naturally and spontaneously to a music therapist now and then, I do not think their constant use fits into the kind of tuning and flow that can be so helpful for relating to the average hospitalised patient. That the analytical music therapist can think in this way and use this as a basis for titled musical improvisations is another matter. However, whether transference interpretations should or should not be used by an analytical music therapist is a question that each therapist must answer for himself on the basis of personal experience, experimentation, and observation of results under expert supervision.

Having made my point about the difference between the therapist's distortional transference and e-countertransference, I will, in the rest of the book, revert to the usual term countertransference so as not to burden the student with a term not at present in general use.

Essay Ten

Survival

As far as he is in control of the matter, the therapist owes it to his patients to survive. The hospitalised patient did not survive, at least temporarily, she succumbed to psychiatric illness. But the therapist tries to offer a new model for coping with stress. He must survive being the bearer of the projections and penetrations by projective identification of his patients, without himself identifying with them. He must survive to challenge the omnipotence of his patients' destructive impulses and phantasies. These may have appeared to damage their real parents in the past, but should now leave their therapist/parent reasonably resilient and imperturbable. He must survive the rejection that is his patients' way of communicating the hurt caused by her being, or feeling she was, rejected by parents, friends, lovers, life---or ultimately herself.

He must survive filling his mind with the strange images from his patient's unconscious, as he recreates their dreams and visualisations in his own mind; and filling his ears with rhythmic patterns of anxiety, hate, fear and terror, also at times when his own life rhythms are less than bouyant. He must survive the often difficult conditions of work in institutions through impoverished times, with inadequate or unsuitable premises, unspeakable pianos, a painful lack of equipment and a minimum establishment of hours to integrate fully with the team as well as aiming at proving his worth in his contact work.

If this sounds a depressive view of psychiatric music therapy then I have succeeded in my aim. It can be and has been like this. But since I have retired I have seen music therapy departments spring up in other areas which offer a different picture, with geographical space for storage of instruments and timespace for the therapists' recovery from stressful contact work. All this is not to say, however, that this work cannot offer rich rewards and marvelous shared creative experiences for both therapist and patient in between all the struggle. It can and does. But that is all the more reason for examining the conditions necessary for the therapist's survival.

I think this chapter is the examination of the shadow side of the remark that so many people have made to me and many of my colleagues on hearing that we were music therapists i.e. "Wonderful work you are doing, wonderful work." Of course this is preferable to the other common remark: "What on earth is music therapy?" But if he only stays with the wonderful work view of things the music therapist may feel increasingly guilty and perplexed if he finds himself suffering from fatigue, disillusionment, fading ideals, and becomes ultimately burnt-out and drops out.

Let us look at some of the facts. Those working in psychiatric hospitals have a considerably higher rate of suicide or breakdown than do average citizens. Psychiatrists, for example, have almost the highest suicide rate of any profession. Medical doctors have twice the national average suicide figure. It is arguable that people are drawn to these professions for unhealthy reasons and that their suicide rate is higher because they have access to drugs and know the lethal doses. I do not know whether the first thesis is true, but the second surely is.

However, I do know from twenty years of experience, that at first even our buoyant young music therapy students, who we supervised during their practical training at the hospital where I worked part-time, were not prepared for the overwhelming fatigue and malaise that they often experienced at the end of a seven-hour working day at the hospital. Later on the work became helpfully interspersed with more staff groups as there was increasing accent on multi-disciplinary teamwork. The general climate today is open to considering that stress as "distress" is something that should be taken into consideration in all professions and is not so much a shame as a problem to be solved.

The music therapist is first and foremost a musician, in Britain he has had many more years in that training working towards his musical diploma than in the therapy training. Most of his earlier hours of learning have been in a one-to-one setting with another musician who is almost always, though not absolutely invariably and sometimes not on the surface, a person of warmth, sensitivity, resonance and of actual geographical physical closeness. That is to say that in all my violin lessons my teachers stood close enough to me to put out a hand and touch me. Whether they did or didn't is not the matter for discussion here, but this is an important point.

Furthermore, having been trained, the musician shares with his audience the emotion with which he has enlivened a composer's music and people clap. The message is: "You have done something for us and now we acknowledge this." There is some reciprocity. Some of my erstwhile colleagues are blase about this, and say that applause is the thing that delays one from getting home for dinner. But when they first try playing cold in a radio recording studio they may agree with me that after all it had been a good starter to the dinner.

The training of medical people, I am assured, is quite different. Faced with dead bodies and off-cuts of former citizens, emotion is the last thing that is encouraged. Strangely enough, being in the business of health, the latter part of their training is arranged in such a manner as to ruin the health of all but the toughest of them by asking them to work as many hours in a week as a widowed mother of newborn twins and six other children. It seems that approval and the need for it are considered to be a suspicious sign of dependency and immaturity and so it is witheld from almost every one almost all the time by almost everyone else. Perhaps if it were not, we might have had more co-operation from the cleaners and other members of hospital staff.

Another little warning on the shadow side, is that as a newly-admitted music therapy student, one may have a vision of oneself and all the noble team of therapists extending their role as healers and carers to all those who need or deserve such attention other than their patients---such as their colleagues when in distress. In fact, this is not always the case, and the reverse can sometimes be expected. When the store of warm, positive regard wears thin one must not be surprised at being treated as an emotional lavatory by the best of healers or therapists. However, I must admit that when it was me that was guilty of the behaviour that comes with stress and exhaustion, it was only then that I truly discovered the personally-unique healing qualities of each of my colleagues. Healers and hedgehogs---is the one the other inside out?

A second difference between the musical and medical worlds that struck me, was that in the psychiatric hospital we heard so much about teamwork. I never heard this phrase used in my orchestral days, though looking back I am not certain that I ever knew what the Danish word for teamwork was. It seemed that with music the achievement of a magnetic feeling of unity was much more possible and prevalent in an orchestra than in the hospital. I suppose it helps to have your part written out before you. You never get the oboe player coming along and saying,"I think I will play those four bars of solo there" or come to rehearsal to find the cellist sitting in your place. So it can be upsetting at first to find that your long-awaited individual session is interrupted by someone calling for your patient to do her washing-up which is on the rota, or to arrive in good time and wait endlessly for the patient you have had expensive supervision on only to find that she has been herded off to see the planes grounded in the fog at the local airport. However, when your rage has subsided these things can be sorted out if you can find the time for the meeting of all concerned. One misses the conductor, I suppose. So when the music therapist is disillusioned by the notion of teamwork in his hospital, let him go back to the concert hall and hear a great symphony concert or a fine chamber orchestra. Such musical teamwork can be a great inspiration.

As trainee music therapists most of us are newcomers to the medical world though many medical people themselves are happy and active in the area of music, whether active or passive. For us senior members of the profession our brush with hospitals has often been early and extremely traumatic. For me entrance into these halls of scientific learning and practice still resonates with real horror and terror, only alleviated slightly by being paid for being there or as a visitor trying to desensitise myself by eating the grapes of my rehabilitating relatives.

However, many of my young colleagues take delight in the psychiatric medical world, the jargon, the procedures, the interesting new drugs and approaches, and the creative therapies, and the real teamwork that they find no difficulty in locking into is a pleasure to them. But for those who do not feel like that, I would advise to remember that you were first and foremost a musician probably attracted to the profession by the beauty of sounds and lovely rhythms and the tender, tough and triumphant emotions expressed through them; and though we do still meet monstrous psychically-formed turtles and rhinoceri in the medical profession, some of them, at least, were once attracted to the work by the beauty of the harmonious rhythms of the healthy human body.

The former therapists have no need to read on, but the others have need of a strong, inner sense of personal value and for the value of their work. How can this be achieved? In answer to this I would go back to the therapist's first occupation. He is, as I said, first and foremost a musician. But during our long training it is possible that music has become for him a task, a manner of earning his bread and paying the electricity bill, a subject with which to try and penetrate the unfeeling skulls of restless, frustrated schoolboys barnacle-encrusted with knowledge and saddened with endless sitting indoors with the sun outside seemingly shining for nothing.

Then let him go back to the music that led him into this strange medical world and sustain him. Let him experiment with it as the sacred and healing art that it is. Let him be both a performer at concerts, however minor, and a listener who can appreciate what great interpretive artists have created out of their more one-pointed lives. Let him keep fresh the excitement of new or previously unknown music along with new interpretations of old favourites.

At the hospital where I worked for twenty years, Peter Wright, one of the three original Intertherapy companions and a fine pianist and explorer of lesser known psychic regions, initiated a quarterly concert in the large ecumenical church in which two of the four in our department performed on a rota basis one or two movements of a major work, usually a concerto. On top of this he, himself, performed in a quarterly solo piano recital as a personal challenge and a public sharing of his love of music with patients and staff. Such concerts helped to keep up our standards of performance and to refute the irksome saying that performers who fail become teachers who fail, who become music critics who fail, who become music therapists.

We performed concertos by Brahms, Schumann, Bach, Rachmaninoff, Mozart and Vivaldi, among others. After the last concert, one of my severely ill manic-depressive patients, in a depressive phase, had hardly been able to speak at all in her sessions but after we had improvised together she remembered the concert and asked me to thank the whole department for the lovely music.

Chamber music, performed for the love of it, can be a truly enriching experience and a suitable antidote to all the depression and bitterness fed into the therapist during an average working week. I would especially recommend the eighteenth century composers with their sense of balance, ease and joy. To set the mind to recreating such beautiful forms is to regain the sense of the value of beauty and harmony as something worth striving for and receiving with appreciation when it appears unexpectedly. With regard to this I have never noticed such magnificent sunsets as on those Thursday evenings at the hospital when we were hurrying, heavily laden with instruments, to the last ward session of the week.

Choirs, too, are lovely things to get lost in when the work is over, becoming a vibrant part of a great sonic body and losing one's narrow identity with its psychic bruises and strains. Even analysts are not proof against such ills. In a letter to me the eminent Jungian analyst and writer Dr. Gerhard Adler wrote, "No evening, after work, is possible to me without listening to music."

Yes, sometimes listening is what one wants if one does not care to be active. One can have a very decided opinion of what music is needed to fill the empty places. Sometimes, as with certain kinds of food, I will take a piece of music and hear it over and over again for a few days. Then it will have done its work, I will have absorbed its musical vitamins and want something different. Most people use music in this way without necessarily thinking of it as therapy. For the music therapist who works mostly actively with music, a little awareness of what music he is wanting when at home, and when and how it is effecting him is, in itself, a useful study.

For some time I used to relax regularly to a piece of Turkish music on cassette which had a steady "Ta-tate-Ta-Ta" rhythm. I went deeper and deeper into relaxation until the memories of early traumas locked into my muscles and nervous system started to release themselves physically. I found this rather unsteadying to experience alone and after a while went into holistic therapy to sort out these body memories in a more physical way. Another of these cassettes, based on ancient Sufi tunes, started in restless seven in a bar time and seemed to collect all the restlessness inside me and then broke into a wonderfully soothing four in a bar. That one was for the liver, the blood and for peace. When you are dealing with the deep struggle with difficult emotions with patients these steady rhythms are often more soothing than 19th century symphonic music. Many music therapists doing psychiatric work have said the same.

Almost any activity is recreative if it loses in you the sense of passing time and brings a powerful and reassuring sense of the eternal now. Activities done hurriedly and with irritation, because half your mind is wanting to do something else, are energy-consuming in a deleterious way. Curiously enough I find shopping for more than one day's supply of food very cleansing to the mind. Either operating in an outdoor market where the vitality and wit of the stallholders, the Breughel atmosphere of life in all its variety provide a powerful life-enhancing music of its own, or wielding a mean trolley in Adagio and Prestissimo in the supermarket can be a good mind-clearer, with a champion snooker player's fine geometric calculations. Other people will find their recreation environments elsewhere, in small boats, on river banks, in sports halls, in love. Anywhere which cleanses you of the cobwebs.

After some very disturbing sessions with psychotic patients, meditation is very steadying, even if only practised on the tube on the way home. This may seem rather rarified in contrast to the answer given by a group of art and music therapists to the question: "What restores you best after a hard day's therapy?" "Food!" they roared.

The music therapy novice may make the mistake of bringing home all the problems of his work and mulling them over, anxiously wishing that he had done this or avoided that. This is especially common where there is not a large caseload. He has to realise that he did an hour's work as well as he could and he cannot do more until the next session. Of course he must seek advice if he genuinely feels that a case presents problems which he is too inexperienced to face alone. Some therapists find a regular supervision session alone or with a group of colleagues, or even a interdisciplinary case supervision group, to be a great help, not only with their own professional problems but in realising that others, further along the path, are not ashamed to air their doubts and uncertainties. Working alone, initially, he will be at the mercy of his blind spots.

The therapist will always experience most stress in working with patients who are freely expressing impulses that he himself is repressing. There may then be a tendency to project these on to the patient so that he identifies soley with his own super-ego. In this way he could act in a harsh and anti-therapeutic way or in not doing so he might be worn down by his inner conflict.

Ideally, the music therapist should consider embracing the opportunity to teach as well as learn, as soon as he can. This prevents staleness, rekindles enthusiasm and clarifies his thoughts. I believe that it is very important for an analytical music therapist to attend to this balance in his functions. This profession can exercise the emotional side more than the thinking side most of the time for many of us, therefore verbal groups for supervision, case discussion and problem-solving create a healthy balance to the constant spontaneous expression of emotion that this music demands. There is nothing against congenial groups for "ridding the psyche of accretions of stimuli" either, whether or not eating and drinking are part of that programme. The psychiatric world can be painfully solemn, pompous and dry, and we musicians have to laugh sometimes, otherwise how can our spirits keep light enough to play Mozart and Debussy?

Music therapy is, basically, about tuning another human being, as carefully and painstakingly as one tunes one's violin before playing the simplest melody. Sometimes one tunes to another instrument of standard pitch and sometimes---often in hospital---one must tune one's violin down to a piano as much as half a tone flat and play Mozart's sonata in A in G sharp major. (Pity the violinist with perfect pitch who can be utterly confused in his dual awareness of the keys). The same variation is necessary in tuning patients. I like one of the Hasidic sayings in Martin Buber's "Ten Rungs" (1947) which I think is relevant here: "If you want to raise a man from mud and filth, do not think it is enough to stay on top and reach a helping hand down to him. You must go all the way down yourself, down into the mud and filth. Then take hold of him with strong hands and pull him and yourself up in to the light" (p. 84-85). And there you are, proud and smiling but nevertheless covered in mud and badly out of tune. So an important part of the music therapist working in psychiatry is keeping the instrument of his own self in tune. How he does this is a very individual matter but here are a few suggestions.

He can have a beautiful object---a flower, painting, sculpture or such thing---in his place of work and steal a few seconds now and then to accept its harmony. (Incidentally it marks an important moment in the development of awareness and gratitude in his patient when she, one day, notices it too and speaks appreciatively about it).

Of course, it is not strictly speaking necessary to have an external object, but an internal object is more difficult to share.

He can try to reorient himself in a different room and atmosphere for some minutes in between sessions. Twice a day he can create for himself a period of recreation when he uses his body, preferably outside. This does not necessarily mean that he need be playing badminton or chasing butterflies, it is more that he approaches this period of time, be it half an hour or less, with a different attitude. It is playtime, for the mind, the imagination, the hands, anything that will help him to feel more alive and refreshed. It sounds easy but it takes a serious intention to pull that time out of the hurrying stream of the daytime hours.

I would suggest that two days a week are kept free from therapy, though he may well find that he has reports to write or professional meetings to attend. These two days should preferably be consecutive as it is only on the second day that one really achieves a gentler and more bouyant rhythm in the inner music. Ideally one weekend a month could be spent away from home if he lives in a big city, in congenial surroundings with good friends or in a more stimulating atmosphere if he lives in a country backwater. I recommend this after only having achieved it during six months of my music therapy life following a major operation. I felt so extraordinarily well and relaxed on the Monday following that weekend that I vowed I would make it a regular practice. Did I? Well, guess when I wrote this?

It is a temptation to take the holiday allowance here and there, as circumstances permit. But I really would recommend the three or four weeks in a row as there is a cumulative deepening of relaxation followed by space for new ideas and enthusiasm for the work to be done. Apart from holidays, the music therapist working in psychiatry will have to keep to a life-style which will enable him to do his work. What was a fitting life style for a performing or even teaching musician may not be right for the music therapist. Personally I need periods of solitude in which to sink down into a well of tranquility within myself. If I do not have these I find it difficult to make emotional contact with the patients and I have scant access to counter-transference which feels like having a perceptive organ removed. It has been an experience that I wish to avoid. However, apathy is also to be avoided. One needs stimulation when one has the energy to enjoy it. It is a matter of balance on a razor-edged path.

I was surprised and worried to find that an excess of exogenous joy put me temporarily out of tune with my hospital patients. I had to return quietly to some inner midpoint before I could be in touch with them again. I am ashamed to say that the week before my holiday I was filled with a most urgent desire to get away from the pressures and burdens of work and I found it a great struggle to stay carefully tuned to my patients' emotional levels. After a holiday, too, it was difficult to adjust, but one did so more willingly. However, therapists vary over this. When I was in analysis I found the first session after the holiday was a dead session but the last one before the holiday was unusually stimulating, giving me plenty to think about. These difficulties in adjustment are seldom mentioned in connection with therapy, as tutors themselves have often not had such experience and therefore the new music therapist can feel very guilty and inadequate when he runs up against them for the first time and thinks he must be the only person who ever felt like this.

Perhaps the most insuperable barriers to harmonious therapy, from the music therapist's point of view, are serious long-term problems within his own co-resident family, or, with younger therapists, the less than successful pursuit of the much-desired beginnings of a family unit. Such difficulties which continue through the weekend, the night and what should be the holidays, can gradually exhaust the music therapist more completely than dealing with patients who are handing him back their life's damage. Work can become the escape of a work-aholic, and then the dissonances rise to the surface of his mind again when he gets home, to erode the renewal of his vitality. I mentioned this to two Intertherapy students, one of whom did have family problems and said to me, "What are you supposed to do? Get rid of the family?" One cannot plaster a label on one's nearest and dearest marked "Not wanted on voyage!" But one can be aware of the danger of letting an emotionally draining situation continue untreated and not be too proud to reach out for any help that is available for dealing with it.

Another situation to avoid, I agreed with Freud about this, is treating people pushed unwillingly into therapy with you by their relations. It seldom works. They are not really motivated themselves and personally I find the "prophet-is-not-honoured-in-his-own-country" syndrome rather confidence-eroding. It is also better, I believe, to have other people treat your nearest relatives. I think a mother's job is to be a mother and a husband's to be a husband. A certain coldness creeps in when one is treating those bound by love with clinical thinking. However, Little Hans (Freud 1909 Vol.X) could have been an exception to this rule though we never heard the rest of the story of that family. So I am not sure that this applies to small children.

Finally, a word or two about success and failure. One must take the long-term view. There is a very wise passage in the Tao Te Ching which runs: "For things sometimes go forward, sometimes they lag behind; sometimes they breathe gently, sometimes they pant violently; sometimes they are strong, sometimes they are feeble; sometimes they start afresh, sometimes they decay. Therefore the saint avoids too much emphasis; he avoids extravagance; he avoids excess." Not that the therapist is a saint, we covered that in the Wonderful Work bit. However, failure can seem to lurk in events which turn out well later on: patients who test us by staying away or coming late, or patients who leave only to do better with our colleagues, or patients who clutch on to their secondary gains and make no progress at all until we set a date for their departure. But whatever one reckons as failure, it sticks in one's mind like a thorn and can teach us a great deal when at last some useful conclusion has been extracted from it.

Success, too, can bring its problems, especially if the people working with the patient are not a team, meeting together at least occasionally. But what can we call success? There are little sparks of it all along the road if one is alert to them, and it is great to be able to share them with colleagues. Sometimes one works with patients who evince a veritable transformation. Not often, but when it happens it can be very beautiful, like freeing a bird which flies with its own effort up into the fresh air and sunlight. It makes one feel very humble. One did so little and yet... But with the team, if there is not too much envy around, one can celebrate. For these moments alone the struggle for survival as a therapist in a psychiatric hospital is very much worthwhile.

And lastly, the shock of a patient who kills herself. Naturally one will examine one's work to see if one could have done more to prevent it. But the burden of the death rests broadly on the patient's environment, both past and present, the team, the therapist and the patient herself. Although it can be a devastating experience, the therapist hopefully will not feel too much guilt. Such an action is always a harsh blow to all who were involved with the patient and often it leaves much residual anger which may initially hide the sorrow for a wasted life.

People vary enormously in their toleration of stress as distress. It partly depends on resonances from the past, and partly on the "tough and tender mindedness" of the therapist. Sometimes the careworker survives but their family takes the stress. Therefore each therapist must find his own blueprint for survival. I wrote this chapter hoping that it might give some budding music therapists in trouble with feeling that they did not feel wonderful about their "wonderful work" the incentive to "live empirically" as Jung suggested.

If the discussion in this chapter has no meaning for you and paints a gloomy picture of your happy therapy position, then the world has moved on and thank goodness for that.

Essay Eleven

Music Therapy and Love

This essay is included because of the danger, in the techno-logical and analysing climate of today, of forgetting the value of the "heart" qualities of compassion and empathy. Many of us remember being put off a subject in school by a cold, unfeeling teacher. Later in life this could have been regretted as it might have been the foundation of a useful and necessary branch of learning. The same thing can happen in therapy though it is understood that astringency and rigor also have their place, but mostly with regard to the therap-ist's attitude to his own work and the keeping of boundaries rather than in his attitude to the patient.

Chambers' 20th Century Dictionary defines love as "to regard with benevolence." This sounds to me to be a weak and passive kind of love, and I prefer the Chinese definition of Jen in the ancient Confucian commentary: "Jen is to love men joyously and from the innermost of one's heart." It sounds robust and active and capable of giving happiness to both the giver and the recipient. Naturally, Jen here means mankind rather than the male sex only. A more modern definition appears in "The Road Less Travelled" (1983) by the Christian psychiatrist Dr. M. Scott Peck. He defines love as: "the will to extend one's self for the purpose of nurturing one's own or another's spiritual growth." Here we have the idea of loving oneself as well as others, which brings us to the biblical command to "Love your neighbour as yourself."

But there is no loving of self or others without oneself having been loved first. To love one's neighbour as oneself (or anyone else) one has first to have been loved in a way that one's physical needs of food and warmth were met and one's feelings were understood and one's true self respected, not perfectly understood and respected but at least "well-enough" as described by Winnicott (1965).

Therapy is about this special way of loving, and music therapy offers the additional dimension of subverbal communication with loving meetings via sound patterns. The therapist offers a maternal holding to the client. He improvises reflectively on the more primitive themes offered to him, meanwhile mirroring her emotions as a good mother might. In the music the therapeutic couple can partly revive the memories of the emotion and kinaesthetic awareness surrounding the preverbal communication of the earliest stage of life, with its mysterious loving and incubating qualities.

In real life, loving takes different forms at different periods of life. First there is the symbiotic love of mother and infant, essential for life in its earliest stage but stifling if kept on at a later stage. This produces the primary narcissism and healthy delight-in-self of the young child which is the basis of self-esteem throughout life.

Next comes the reciprocal love of friends, it may have been this kind of love that Freud was describing when he said that along with the exigencies of life, love is the greatest educator; and it is through the loving actions to those nearest to him that the incomplete human being is taught to respect its laws and so avoid the punishments following on the neglect of them. I think the reader would enjoy reading the original text either in translation or in Freud's German mother tongue. (See Volume 14 of his Complete Works, p. 312).

Later on comes the genital love which may set in train lifelong responsibilities and commitments. Lastly there is the protective and nurturing love of parents, teachers and therapists, the last-named two sometimes having to make up for omissions in the love of the first-named; or the denied shadow side of a defensively idealised parent.

There can easily be an imbalance in the love of self and love of neighbour and, curiously enough, I have found in my analytical music therapy practice that most of my clients needed help in being able to love themselves. For example, a young student came to me saying that he used all his leisure time being involved in political activities. After 12 sessions he came to see that he was neglecting his own self-development and he decided to spend some time working for a further qualification.

Sometimes the client is trying to love himself in the other. That student was struggling to help the underprivileged working classes instead of giving the underprivileged working-class aspect of himself a chance to develop. Naturally it is not a case of loving either one or the other. He ended up with a better balance between loving himself and his fellowmen.

People in caring professions---teachers, priests, nurses and therapists---to name but a few, very often project their own unhappy "inner child" on to their clients and try to care for it there as was discussed in a previous essay. The result is that their own deprived child self becomes starved, and they often spend more and more of their time on clients to avoid confrontation with this ravenous side of themselves. At the same time they can feel totally depleted by certain clients.

In analytical music therapy we help them to regain their inner child by improvising musically as their client, pupil or parishioner, with all her pain and distress. Spending time and loving attention on the ensuing emotions in the sessions can gradually help to gain awareness of and then heal the hurt and free more energy for daily life.

A paediatrician client from the continent discovered that she was projecting her inner child on to her little patients; and then found it so difficult to communicate with them that she almost came to hate them. Tracing the lost and unhappy child part of herself back through the years, through her music she at last discovered her creative, happy child aspect. She played a lovely, lively improvisation, playing first a rather rigid doctor and then the bouncing, lilting rhythms of the child. This was largely done through the Splitting Technique, in which therapist and client take turns to play two aspects of the client, or the client and another person on to whom she is projecting certain aspects of herself. The client comes to see the other person in a different light and finds out what she is projecting on to this person. This usually makes the subsequent relationship with that individual easier and more realistic. In playing two aspects of herself, the client brings these two sides closer together, so that they can exchange some of their qualities and make a useful cross-fertilisation.

Greater love, of self and life and others, is the ultimate aim of all analytical music therapy, but sometimes one has to discover the hate first. Former Intertherapy student Professor Ole Teichmann- Mackenroth in a letter described how a widowed lady had needed to work through her antagonism towards her late husband before she could admit to the ways in which he had influenced her and she had lovingly followed him; and only then could she complete her mourning process.

For a time I saw a partially autistic man of 24 and his mother. They sat side by side, not touching one another until after the session in which we verbally explored how they behaved when they were angry with one another. At the next session they held hands. The exploration of their negative feelings allowed them to express their love and closeness.

A male client in his sixties expressed a false self who loved his wife in an idealising, passive way but was seething with rebellion unconsciously. Gradually he became able to express this rebellion and could also tolerate his ambivalence to his music therapy, without visibly destroying me, but not yet to his wife. However, he did not know what he wanted out of life, only what he did not want. Until he had worked through his hate and rebellion, he could not love in a creative way.

Love can be compared with a spring of water. Music therapy, like most other therapies, is used to clear away the blockages to the spring; but unlike them, it is also used to express the joy of the spring itself, as was discussed in the essay on celebrations. A psychotherapist friend said he could do this with his clients too, but I am sure there is not the immediacy and internationally understood mutual joyous expression that we can experience in musical improvisation.

A middle-aged woman client expressed verbally and musically her venomous feelings towards her second husband, who had been chosen largely for security reasons. He contrasted unfavourably with her first love-chosen husband, who had died in an accident. She gradually found that in her sadness she needed the physical closeness of her present husband, and from here their sexual relationship revived. Having expressed all the frustration with him, she was surprised to find in him some supportive and amiable sides. Expressing the hate freed some love to flow.

A young wife and mother had always been frigid sexually. After discovering delights in sound improvisation, she drew a picture of animals in pens representing her sexual libido. She then improvised on the picture imagining freeing these animals. After nineteen sessions she found a formerly unexperienced delight in sexuality. However, until we had worked on the oedipal transference on to her husband, these joys did not include him.

In the dyadic improvisation there can be a loving that allows the client to be, that enfolds her with appropriate sound or challenges her to be herself and show her real feelings. There can be warm, reciprocal sharing of feelings---no cold Freudian mirror here. The improvisation can be (but is not necessarily) an expression of true feelings which can be put outside the self and thus shared. In order to do this there must be trust, which is part of love, on the part of the client; and some giving of psychic space by the therapist. This is another kind of love, a listening love, a resonating love, a maternal Yin kind of love that is a giving of permission to be.

I say that music is not necessarily the expression of true feelings because of some work I did with a young schizophrenic woman. Theresa presented with two personalities; subsequently there were four. There was a high, flat-voiced conventional personality that she took on when with her mother and at first with me. Also a disjointed, emotional and deeper-voiced personality which she began to take on when the therapy was going well. Her improvisation was straight out of No. 1 personality and a real negation of feelings. At the fourth session she asked me what sort of a girl I saw her as and I told her about the two personalities. She managed to express them in music with the second one, though extremely short, being much more lively, spontaneous and imaginative. Through this improvisation she managed to be more loving to herself in allowing a deeper musical expression to be shared. At first she was given a space to fill but had a terrible fear of filling it with her true feelings for fear of rejection.

As the therapist I find that love is an essential ingredient in the therapy. The client's transference love for the therapist enables her to struggle to overcome her weaknesses and eventually to find subsititute love objects in the world outside, where the boundaries do not preclude the physical development of expression. The therapist's love for the client aims at being not a sentimental or smothering love but a true empathy, enabling him to see life as much from the point of view of the client as possible; but at the same time not to lose his own orientation. It is very difficult to work with a client effectively before this balance of love is established.

On the other hand, the therapist's love for himself and caring for himself are important as they make it unnecessary to project his own inner child on to the client while starving himself of loving care. Not to allow the client to intrude unnecessarily into the time outside the hour, requires a special sort of loving from the therapist, and creates a special more mature form of loving in the client. There is a balance of respect and love. The therapist respects his client's ability to contain her feelings just that bit more than she thought she could and to reach out into the world for what she is missing in the therapeutic relationship; and the client respects her therapist's frail humanity.

The client's love for her therapist does not exclude hate. Love and hate are two poles of one continuum. They do not cancel one another out; each exists in its own place. Perfect love may cast out fear but it does not cast out hate, which is the negative aspect of love. Alexander Lowen expresses this as two concentric circles with love in the inside guarded by hate (1965).

The therapist's love for the client can be a shield. A client, remembering her dead father, first recalled his strictness over her faulty piano-playing and his beatings. Then she wept when she remembered thinking that if she now performed well enough in concerts, perhaps he somehow would hear her. The therapist, who had recently lost his own father, was able to hold the client in loving concentration and was thus enabled to look away from his own sorrow and focus wholly on her during the session. But after the session he felt quite depressed on his own behalf, and shed tears.

Loving can be holding someone close, physically and emotionally, but it can also be letting go. As parents of adolescents gradually let their child go, the therapist gradually lets the client go and the client gradually lets the therapist go as she reaches out to the life outside the session. Any kind of holding on or holding back here smacks of lack of trust on the part of one or other of the parties and is indicative of lack of a greater and more all-embracing love. Of course, there are plenty of difficullties on the way, but loving is toleration of the chaos that precedes creativity. It is daring to discover the hidden treasures in the heart of the client and oneself as therapist, even though they are guarded by the symbolic monsters of fairy tales.

A special kind of love by the music therapist is the love of music. Not just the polished pearls of composed music of the masters but the ability to clothe all shades of emotion in a musical form. This can be a wonderful freedom and a delight to him; having an intimate, non-verbal, musical exchange---with clients who may have aphasia, mental handicap, physical disability, catatonic states or even crippling shyness---can be a richly rewarding experience for both of them.

The contrast between the clinical, measurable side of music therapy seen in research figures and the immeasurable waywardness of love, is great, and may necessitate achieving a delicate balance in the future. But it will always be essential to keep both in mind in order to understand the positive results of music therapy.

Essay Twelve

The Place of Structure
In Musical Improvisation

At first glance it may seem strange that there should be any talk of structure in connection with something as free as musical improvisation. This activity appears to give the performer the perfect chance to eschew all kinds of discipline and indulge soley in releasing spontaneity and self-expression. But a second thought will lead us to the realisation that the fact of the expression attaining musical form means that a structure has been imposed on the emotion that gave birth to the musical sounds.

Curiously enough, there is no structure more rigid than the musical form that a patient who knows nothing about music will impose on herself in improvisation. It has the unchanging characteristics of a person's hand writing or rhythmic gait, (though not as unchanging as their finger prints) and it is as uniquely individual. Undoubtedly it is a valid musical form for such a patient's main psychic attitude but it can also have the quality of a straight-jacket.

This reminds us of the strange fact that people faced with complete freedom from some past-imposed discipline usually proceed to write their own Book of Leviticus to give themselves the security of the structure, sense of direction and identity that they have lost.

The aim of the therapist then is not to remove all structure but to replace a crippling structure with a benign enabling one. The structure of the same weekly hour and place, the same instruments, therapist, and the same transaction of exchanging the patient's money for this hour of time and attention, will all be freely accepted by the client. This can be likened to the firm holding that a mother gives to her baby to allow him to feel safe enough to reach out and explore the world. The patient will need to grow and change, and probably experience pain as well as joy in the process; and this holding structure is both a strength and a comfort to her, producing a powerful rhythm in her life.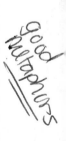

The musical structure as regards rhythm and pitch (less so timbre and dynamics which are more responsive to the mood of the moment) is governed by that mental institution or function which rules the patient's psyche at the time. For example, a thirty-two-year-old schizophrenic man accompanied his deep and mysterious inner imaginings with taut, tonal, somewhat repetitive rhythmic phrases, which every now and then he would alter by changing into another rhythm. This music was expressing the synthetic or synthesizing function of carefully balancing and holding together his lately disintegrated psyche. As we worked together over eighteen months, inklings of expressive feeling: sadness, tenderness and anger filtered through; but still the main function expressed was the synthetic and I did not feel it was right to interfere with this musical expression of his naturally self-healing process in any way.

Another patient, a twenty-four-year-old girl with anxiety neurosis and conversion symptoms, played with great rapidity and always on the xylophone. I had trouble in keeping up with her, and took to playing only interspersed chords as a kind of skeleton behind her clothing semi-quavers. She was expressing the energy of the anxiety behind the symptoms. Sometimes through this expression we would get in touch with some of the phantasies or memories that lay behind the anxiety. As Freud wrote: "Anxiety is therefore the universal current coinage for which any affective impulse is or can be exchanged if the ideational content attached to it is subject to repression" (Volume 16 of the Complete Work, p. 403). And later, he adds that "the generation of anxiety gives place to the formation of symptoms, which results in the anxiety being bound" (p. 405).

In her music the patient as it were unbound the anxiety, being able to tolerate it with the aid of her musical expression. Music being an acceptable activity to the superego, it relaxed its hold on the repressed ideational content from time to time to allow us to see some of the generators of the anxiety behind her symptoms.

Another patient was a 27-year-old man with manic-depressive illness. He started his treatment just as his manic phase was fading but he was still feeling rather omnipotent and very denigrating to me. His music expressed this destructive attitude for some time. He whacked away at the xylophone and drum in a manner which made it very difficult for me to play creatively, apart from the fact that he produced in me a countertransference of crippling uselessness. Later on, when he had worked through some of this feeling, he developed a positive mother transference with occasional flashes of negative father transference; and he began truly to relate reciprocally in our music and to take pride in our mutual creation when we heard the tape back. This was an expression of the ego, first as a defence by projection and denigration, and then by sublimation of the instincts, called up by the good feelings of the mother transference.

In this case the musical structure changed considerably as the patient developed; in the first case (of the schizophrenic) the structure remained much the same but the content became deeper; in the second case (of the anxiety neurotic) the patient came to treatment only once a fortnight and although she did quite well in life, she possibly unconsciously did not feel that she had enough containment to enable her to relax her own musical structure.

Although given perfect musical freedom, these three patients were all given the structure of an idea around which to base their improvisation. This gave them an integrating focus which enabled their musical expression to unfold without self-consciousness. Their task was to create some kind of musical order out of the chaos of their feelings. The mental idea provided an ego focus to help them not to be overwhelmed by their unconscious stirrings, which can be very powerful during such dyadic improvisations. One of such ideas (Assagioli, 1965) is to imagine a door in a long, high wall and placing the title of the subject you wish to explore on the door, to open it and see what is the other side. This can reveal valuable but sometimes very abstruse unconscious symbolism. Some more of his given images are the "Cave Mouth in the Jungle Clearing" that is watched from behind a tree and can reveal symbolically the least developed part of the personality; The "Mountain Climb" which can reveal the picture of the patient's life aspirations; and the "Pool in the Meadow" into which the patient looks to discover phantasy images relating to her sexual development. Other subjects come from the problems that the patient brings up in therapy; some of these which spring readily to mind are "Discipline," "Feeling Unwanted," "Meeting a Friend," " My Husband's Partner" (this was jealousy concerned with his lovely young blonde partner), and "Watering the Desert."

Some patients produce factual subjects most of the time and some (20% of my patients in 1979) produce symbolic subjects. Either kind can reveal deep emotion and unconscious attitudes. This kind of structure I would call <u>the structure of thought</u> but this is not the only kind of structure possible in this kind of dyadic improvisation. Another kind, <u>the structure of musical expression</u>, is quite unusual in most forms of musical improvisation; for example the 12-bar harmonic structure of blues jazz; the rhythmic intricacies and the ragas of classical Karnatic Indian music; Steve Reich's repeated phrases in his hypnotic 18-instrument improvisations; or composer Alfred Nieman's strict rules for atonal improvisation (i.e., no common chords, not more than three chromatic notes in sequence and no octaves).

I do not often introduce this kind of musical structure into a patient's therapy for the reason that it leads the mind away from their feelings and the images from the unconscious, which make up the material with which we work. However, sometimes this musical structure can partly take the place of the ego's synthetic function, and I can give an example of a case in which it was most successful. The thirty-two-year-old man, who I mentioned earlier, habitually used his music to express his synthetic funtion. We were approaching a phase in his therapy when he was beginning to talk a little about the breakdown of his marriage, which actually coincided with his breakdown in health. As we were also at the beginning of his two week holiday, I suggested that we take the title "Separation," which might possibly bring up other separations in his life. We used, for the first time, an Indian raga called the Saraswati raga. I changed the xylophone notes round so the raga formed the natural scale and the patient decided to vocalise and play the xylophone while I played the piano with one line only. The effort needed for him to sing and play in this unusual scale seemed to cause the synthetic function to be allowed partly to be relegated to the actual raga, so that some genuine expression of sadness could be heard in the music, especially in his vocalisation, which at that time usually tended to be rather expression-less and matt, though later it became surprisingly sonorous and expressive. (The scale is C major with F sharp replacing F natural and B flat replacing B). After we had played, he said that he thought first of momentary absences in conversation, then of the people who came and went at work, and lastly of the separation from his divorced wife that had taken him fourteen months to be spoken about. This tolerance of some mourning allowed the patient to talk, for the first time, of the second half of his life and to fantasise fetching colourful bales of cloth and perfumes by boat from Greece (where he had lived and was married) as if allowing some of the richness of that era to enter into his now rather emotionally-impoverished life. The next week he imagined exchanging them all for food, especially fruit, which seemed to express his need now for comfort and stability, in the 6/8 motion of the boat, rather than glamour and sex.

It is as if the super-ego, which does not approve of certain emotions, and demands that they are repressed, approves of a set task, such as playing in a certain scale or mode; and when this is done, the repression is slightly lifted to allow some expression of a formerly intolerable emotion. The scale or mode almost takes the place of the repression.

Apart from suggesting the occasional use of a mode or scale, I have not used the structure of musical form in improvisation, though I know that my colleague Professor Johannes Eschen used to use the rondo form in group improvisation with good results. That is not to say that patients' improvisations do not naturally fall into known musical forms, particularly the ternary (ABA) and less often the binary (AB) forms which one often finds in old dances. But these are not forms which I have imposed from without, they have just been the natural expression of an inner need for this kind of balance to contain the player's expression.

On the whole, unless patients are playing the piano, which is unusual, or the melodica, they play a unilinear melody on the xylophone and it is up to the therapist to harmonise it in the way he thinks best. The harmonic structure is, of course, imposed on the patient, who has no control over it. I tend to use atonal dissonances when I feel that the patient is strong enough to be stimulated to bring out her emotion more forcefully, and to use tonal harmonies where I feel that there is a need to contain emotion in a reassuring way, or to help a fragile patient to tolerate just a little emotion. This, however, does not take into account working with the patient's counter-transference which might demand that one played tonal sadness or atonal madness at a certain time in order to make a patient, who was ready for it, aware of this hidden layer in herself.

Another structure which is useful in dyadic improvisation is the limitation of a certain time span. I used to begin a certain patient's session with a ten minute improvisation. We were quite free as far as subject matter was concerned and there were no musical constraints, but the realisation that the time was limited made him pour his expression into the time available.

Given the boundaries of a structure, people are motivated to see if they can function in spite of them. There is something to pit their strength against and they mobilise all available forces to this end. Even with a totally free dyadic improvisation, each has the restraining factor of the other's dynamics and musical ideas. (This brings to mind those stories of physically-handicapped individuals who perform amazing feats such as the one-legged young man who recently climbed a mountain). With patients, their aggression can be mobilised in the service of expression as a form of self-assertion. This is most valuable and in fact one sees that this happens in the work of all great instrumental performers.

In contrast to this use of structure, I believe that total freedom is a stress in improvisation as well as in life. Faced with total freedom, the patient is subjected to her own possibly very harsh and restricting superego boundaries in expression which she has to impose on her music. This gives her two tasks: creating a structural boundary to suit the harsh supergo and finding some expression through the resulting music. This reminds me of a report of a children's home where the children were brought up totally freely and without restrictions. After some time all the children were found to be anxious and neurotic. When their leaders resorted to more old-fashioned methods of firm boundaries, rules and restraints, their charges settled down and no longer showed such disturbance.

It seems that when a certain structure is advocated in analytical music therapy, it allows the patient a superego cleavage (Waelder 1939) whereby she accepts the boundary of a given structure as a partial superego, releases her own hold on some of the repressed material and allows this to surface in her mind during the improvisation with or without it being expressed in the music. It is also possible and interesting to speculate (though scarcely relevant to this book) that the tenets and boundaries of certain religious sects, that appear so restrictive from the outside, could offer their adherents greater freedom of self-expression than their members might enjoy if they were busy dictating their own private or family self-punitive ten or one hundred and ten commandments.

But to return to music therapy, we sometimes use an improvisation called "Being at the Centre of the World," in fact I think we mean the universe but the world sounds more familiar and less formidable. In this exercise the patient plays quite alone without any musical structure or structure of time, but she has the one thought structure of being alone at the very centre of all that is in the created world. Most patients, and therapists who have tried this, are almost paralysed with awe and scarcely able to play at the beginning of the exercise. Sometimes the patient will start with a thunderous aggressive salvo only to realise that no one else is going to retaliate or even respond because she is the only one who is there. Then there is awe and even sadness. It is a wonderful exercise for a therapist to do before taking a difficult group, after this exercise one is so thankful for any response however violent the attack. However, even this exercise is not really totally free because there is the structure of the idea of "total freedom" and also the projections bouncing off the therapist, possibly as a disapproving super-ego.

Some of the richest phantasies have been experienced using the structure of a very regular rhythm; some of the wildest music has been produced using the structure of a prescribed thought or idea; some of the most elusive repressed emotion has seeped out using the structure of a difficult scale.

The task of the music therapist is to steer a path between no matrix for expression and a structure that is crippling rather than enabling. This is extremely difficult but the successful solution will always be something that offers a degree of satisfaction to super-ego, ego and id and to the synthetic function which achieves a healthy balance between the three. The easier this is for the patient, the less she will find freedom a stress, but until that time comes we must appreciate and value the use of structure in analytical music therapy.

Essay Thirteen

The Meaning Of Music

As a musician, the analytical music therapist suffers from the temptation to let the music created by the therapeutic dyad have its own hidden meaning, as Mendelssohn said "too precise for words." But this means that the session can split into two separate parts, and that feelings can either avoid the words and get hidden in the music, or enter the words but leave the music without deeper content. This rather resembles the danger of members of a therapy group meeting outside their session and exchanging all the important information there, so that they then leave the group session empty of any but the most superficial talk.

It can be asked why it is necessary to try to put the meaning of the music into words. Isn't it enough that the feelings have been expressed? Personally I do not think it is. The cathartic release of tension through the music, without knowledge of what the feelings are about, gives temporary relief, but without understanding in words, the tension will mount again leading to the need for further relief without knowledge and so on. It becomes a kind of acting-out, or rather acting-in. In the session the patient will always be avoiding any close scrutiny or reflective thought on the emotional content of the music. In this way it can become a debilitating leakage from the talking part of the session. Once an emotion is clothed in words, they both can become like building blocks that one can play with.

I am not saying that there is always a split between words and music in a session for there can be valuable fertilisation from the one medium to the other, I am only saying that this split is a danger that the therapist must take into account.

I will freely admit that it has sometimes been a tremendous effort for me to attempt to cross the bridge from music to its message in words. Moving from words to music is simple and often a great relief from the tensions inherent in sticking to verbal concepts. But though the relief of musical expression can be enough, temporarily for the id, it is not enough for the ego, which requires clarification and at least an attempt at understanding.

Very often words can take the patient a certain distance and then dry up and can take her no further. Feelings not conscious enough to form words can be expressed in sound, and when the emotion is thus clothed, words are able to take over the expression of the feelings once more.

so true

Music is always an expression of some kind, but sometimes it is the expression of acceptable feelings and at other times it is the expression of a defence against an unacceptable feeling or impulse. Many musicians take up the musical profession because of the opportunity of the relief through expression in sound without the danger that anyone will be able to crack their musical code. That is not to say that there are not some exceptional, fine musicians who can delve into deep feelings through a combination of musical and verbal expression. But it is rare, because words and music are two quite separate languages and the interpreters are few and far between.

Therefore a most important part of the analytical music therapy session is when therapist and patient listen to the playback of the recording of their improvisation. The patient must learn to listen to her music and take the responsibility for what feelings she clearly expresses. She will also, probably for the first time, listen to the interaction of her own and the therapist's music, as most often the patient is oblivious of the therapist's music during the actual improvisation, anyway at a conscious level.

The therapist, too, must learn to listen to the music in the patient's voice tones. For example, a patient who had made an unsuccessful attempt at suicide had a high, unreal-sounding voice and seemed to be imagining that she had been successful in the suicide and had found herself to be immortal or at least successful in killing off the feelings of anger and despair which had driven her to try and kill herself in the first place. At the end of the session in which she had expressed some of the murderous rage in musical sounds, her voice was fuller and deeper.

Another woman, not a patient this time, had come back from a holiday abroad with a close family group in which there was mutual support during the slow death of the father of the family. Her voice was full of unusually deep tones from the ability to accept the whole range of emotion in response to this situation with its supportive setting, and from the ability to face and accept at least the external experience of a death among people for whom it meant much the same as it did for her.

A middle-aged woman patient, who lived and worked at home alone, had been having strange feelings in the evening. At first she had been experiencing some depression, then she described the feelings as hysterical, and then they had come round to being anxious. We improvised on the title of "Evening Feelings" and she played a high ostinato note on the xylophone to express her anxiety, and then she played about comforting acts like having a bath, reading a nice book and having a warm drink, all of which finally routed the anxiety. In this way she was able to take over a maternal function to comfort her anxious child feelings but first she had to give them expression which could then be reflected upon.

Another time this same patient, who always played the part of a pleasant, reasonable and rational person, had been watching a television programme about a witch and demon possession. She had found it rather disturbing. We decided to improvise on the theme of going to see a witch and asking her a question. As she played she imagined going forward to a dark presence and being told to work out her next step and not ask any more questions. The music seemed to suggest a child hiding and playing. The witch was the unlovable side of her parents, probably her father who had tossed her a booklet on career opportunities and told her to find herself something to do, leaving her alone to get on with it. Here the child playing in the music gave the clue that the unhelpful witch was the internalised bad aspect of her doctor father whose action had somehow made it impossible for her to get a job suitable to her intelligence and background at any time in her life.

A schizophrenic man was rebuilding his life after a hospital admission. He had formerly studied for one of the professions but was now working in a commercial setting. He had not seen any of his former colleagues but was delighted when one had asked his father where he was. The patient wanted to meet this former friend, and asked that we should improvise a reality rehearsal to prepare him for the meeting. He was afraid of awkward silences and felt that he must have some topics of conversation ready. At first our two parts did not get together in the music, but towards the latter half the music of friendship was weaving in and out gently with some tenderness. I felt that the patient knew what he was working towards.

The next week he came along to his session and said how everything had gone smoothly and what a happy, easy evening it had been. He had not had to work at thinking up topics of conversation, the talk developed fluently and naturally. His music had expressed his fears and then hopes for the evening.

The therapist must remain aware, sensitive and responsive, always ready to react to either the overt or covert feelings which the patient is offering him, though being ready to take his own line when he thinks fit. He must start from a point of emptiness and beware of falling into any set emotional pattern of his own. In actual fact, I think that there is little danger of this for most therapists; but perhaps more danger of sometimes lacking the courage to respond fearlessly to the countertransference feelings that they may receive from patients.

The therapist's music meets the inner pain of the patient with a healing gentleness, or it rages against the world and fate with her in a duet of blinding bitterness. But it is always in tune with the point of greatest sensitivity. In music the therapist says," Yes, I understand, I feel what you feel in this moment" and yet he must not be overcome by these feelings nor locked in alone with them as the patient was. As the therapist plays, the patient is relieved by the sharing of his emotion. The empathy is a fact which can be heard and experienced and received into the patient's empty places inside. It is not just a word which can be denied or disbelieved.

Often the music is "healing" in the sense of making whole a situation which was incomplete where the words left it. A young schizophrenic woman of twenty-seven came to her session saying how various people loved her---her brothers and sister, her ex-husband, her boyfrind and her dead parents. She seemed astonished to find herself so lovable. But there seemed to be other feelings lurking beneath all this delight and astonishment. We improvised on the theme of being lovable and unlovable. The gentle glissandi of being loved alternated with angry pounding on the drum with the intolerable anxiety and frustration of being unlovable. There was far more energy in the anger and frustration of being unloved, and that was pushing the patient into this manic stance of needing to consider herself universally beloved. The fear of being unlovable stemmed from its being seen as the reason for her being abandoned by her mother when she was four years old.

A middle-aged woman had had a father with a very violent nature who had abused her when she was fifteen. She said that she hated him and had always regarded him as wicked rather than sick because she believed that he knew exactly what he was doing. However, there were various pointers towards quite positive feelings for him which were strongly repressed. In our improvisation I did not take the id position (of the positive feelings) to try and force some expression of these, because this would have aroused anxiety; instead I got the co-operation of her ego by suggesting that in the improvisation she should fantasise killing her father. He had, in fact, been dead for over twenty years. (This session was a sequal to one with a dream connected with her father and some ensuing active imagination in which he had suddenly appeared dead). Her music was played on the drum and cymbal but it was not the wild energetic music of anger and annihilation; instead it was extremely heavy as if every stroke cost her a tremendous effort and, in fact, after a short while she had to stop from sheer exhaustion. She had imagined pounding her father to death (how, she didn't know) and had wanted to cut his genitals off but had not had the strength to go on that far. The music brought out the truth (which I did not pass on to her because I did not feel that she was ready to deal with it) that there was a repressed strong loving and sexually validating force working against her conscious negative feelings for her father.

An analytical music therapy student in Intertherapy was working through angry feelings about a former boyfriend who she said, "never gave me much of anything." The student pair decided to improvise to the title "Beating George," but the music was chaotic and arhythmic and suggested evasion and defence rather than a wholehearted angry attack. This student had unconscious omnipotent phantasies of destruction and did not feel it was safe to unleash her aggression even on drum and cymbal. Whenever she wanted to be aggressive she ended up in tears. The music helped to transmute her inability to use aggression freely into useful self-assertion, quite explicit.

Sometimes a patient's music serves as a special sort of defence.

music as an anchor.

It serves a kind of earthing function like the kite-flyer who stands firmly on earth while his kite soars away in the sky. With the music as anchor the consciousness enters strange, not very well-known regions. A lot of primitive music with lively repetitive rhythm is based on this model. This kind of split can also occur when someone is telling their beads, or meditating with a repeated mantra or wazifa which can free up a part of their mind to experience a vision of another kind of inner world most strangely, without the danger of the person reciting it losing his hold on the here-and-now. Moving out of Freudian terminology into "Psychosynthesis" terms, the person can move from an experience of a personal and even collective unconscious to a superconscious realm; but great discipline is needed to move around safely in this area without a teacher, therapist, guru, or murshid to see that one gets safely back to everyday life and experience. The boundaries of time and mind-focussing on titles makes this kind of experience unusual and brief, if experienced, in analytical music therapy.

The man of thirty-three mentioned earlier, formerly having catatonic schizophrenia, always used this kind of very regular rhythmic, tonal pattern for his music. In one session he improvised on "Going to an Island." He came nearly to it in a large sailing boat and saw that it was a deserted island and sailed away. His music, with its regular beat showed nothing but tenacity. In the next session he went to the island again and found a turtle which led him to green palms and a blue and yellow parrot and some natives who were eating fish. He gave some cymbal clashes for the parrot but otherwise did not disturb his beat by a single demi-semi-quaver, although he could afterwards identify the thick-skinned turtle part of himself and the more rarely appearing flamboyant parrot aspect. His regular pattern of music seemed to me to represent his desperate need to hold the different parts of himself together and I did not find it right to interfere with this in any way.

After working for a year he entered a hostel and one evening there was a quarrel between two shouting residents, one of whom pulled out a knife and threatened the other. He told me this with no emotion at all, but his improvisation about it was the most emotional music he had ever played with me. After this he began to entrust a little more emotion to his rigid musical structures and did some lovely free vocal improvisations playing a second part on the xylophone (in the Aeolian mode or pentatonic scale) with me playing on the piano. There was always a strong countertransference feeling of rapture at the time. This kind of feeling is often explained analytically as the "oceanic feeling," a harking back to the experience of the infant at the breast (See Freud's Complete Works Volume 21, p. 64-72). I do not feel wholly convinced by this explanation having had practical breast feeding experience at length with three sons, an occupation which both Freud and Klein only knew about in theory. To me there seemed to be something much more active and purposeful, deliciously greedy and positively joyful going on in our nursery.

Sometimes the music is instrumental in bringing out hidden feelings with remarkable rapidity. The woman of twenty-seven, mentioned earlier, abandoned by her mother at four years, had attempted the abandonment of her own four year old son prior to a suicide attempt following a quarrel and separation from a boyfriend. I saw her after the attempt but I was then away for a week ill. During this week the patient started to scream, apparently without reason, and to disturb her fellow patients. She did not know why she did this. She had been threatened with being put in the locked ward.

At the next session we improvised on the title "Screaming." She started playing some quiet glissandi on the xylophone while I played a catalytic broken major seventh quaver introduction. After some vicious and erratic bangs on the drum and cymbal, the piano played a tender bar and she sobbed, "I want my Mum" several times in a child's voice, ending in a piteous wail absorbed by G-flat chords. She was so pathetic that it crossed my mind to abandon the music and go and put my arm round her but I decided against it as I thought that there would be many people in her life to do that and only me to express the feelings in music so that she could accept them as hers. Then, as if she realised the rightness and reasonableness of what she had said, she banged forcefully, self-righteously on the drum. Again I made an empathic interlude and she finished off by affirming on the drum her need for a mother. The difference in rhythm and timbre of the initial vicious drum beat and the four-square beat after her outburst seemed most striking to me and to other music therapists to whom I played the tape; but an analyst said that he could not discern it. However, he did say that there was no doubt that the music brought out the rapid realisation of her feelings of loss, and following this session there was no more screaming.

The meaning of music is mysterious at best and indecipherable at worst, but it is a study that is well worth while and may help the analytical music therapist very much in the understanding of his patients. It is not at all easy, and does not appear to come naturally to any trained musician but while the therapist is working in this way with patients, it should not be abandoned because of its lack of exactitude. Even small sparks of insight and understanding can be extremely enriching to therapist and patient alike.

Ideally there should be paid time for the therapist to do this part of the work, but in my time there was not. However, things begin to look brighter for the future of all kinds of music therapy research and I watch with admiration as here and there my bright young colleagues sprout Ph.D.s like mushrooms.

Essay Fourteen

The Musical Response

It is impossible to teach a trainee analytical music therapist how to improvise with a patient. The only thing that one can do is to help him to teach himself. This is something that can develop naturally either before his training period, or during this time. What is needed is that he should come to trust in the validity of his own intuition and his natural musical reponse to the patient. He will learn to let reason give way to his spontaneous reply to the immediate situation in their musical relationship. This may include the gentle promptings of the countertransference messages from the patient's unconscious, as well as the difficult predicament of having to be in touch with the external situation at the same time.

In this work there is an external way of relating to the patient, matching her moods and replying to her phrases of melody; and there is an inner way of feeding back to the patient her unconscious feelings as experienced by the therapist in the countertransference. Quite a lot can be said to help a trainee to relate in the outer way but much less in the inner way. Apart from anything else trainees vary a great deal in their responses to countertransference. For some it is a still, small voice which must be listened for with much concentration, whereas with others it is an almost overwhelming emotional force that they must learn to manage in order to keep their emotional balance.

Perhaps a word should be said here about reducing the unnecessary interruptions to one's therapy sessions in the hospital situation as much and as soon as one can. If you find this paragraph unnecessary in your case then read it as history and be thankful. I once saw and empathised with a frantic note on the door a psychotherapist at our hospital who had to share space with other departments. The note was a desperate plea not to be interrupted, and looked like what an art therapy patient might draw when in a state of acute angst. Often when the patient is beginning to make a vital connection or is coming to an important realisation---one that the therapist has been working painstakingly for hours to get---an interruption can be quite a set-back, and can actually cost the hospital many work hours at a point when this can be ill-afforded in both time and money. Helping staff in other disciplines to understand what you are trying to do with "their" patient may entail dropping some of your regular work for a time in order to clarify your therapeutic approach. Some therapists have had success in doing this before they start in a job, but with the rapid turnover of some staff in psychiatric work this has not always been the foolproof answer either. However, progress is being made all the time and when you come across better ways, shout about them.

The first training that a trainee will have, will be learning to improvise by himself. He will learn to tap his own sources of emotion and improvise in every possible mood---joyous, sad, angry, dreamy and so on, just as an actor in training does. There are two practical ways of doing this. One is for him to go to the piano every day right after breakfast, as I did as a student, put the kitchen timer on for a ten minute setting and just play whatever moods that are in him for that timespan. The other way is for him to go out for a walk and create music in his head to everything that one sees: the rhythms of the wind in the trees, animals walking, children playing, old people limping along with sticks, young people in love, allowing everything to arouse the music inside him. In this way he will learn to create an instant channel of expression that will carry any amount of the required emotion without himself losing control of it or being overwhelmed by it. Thus if he expresses sadness, his music may help his patient to contact her frozen areas of sadness, but he himself should have perfectly dry eyes and breathe easily throughout the improvisation. When he has mastered this art he will learn to respond to another person musically, by improvising in duos and later in trios, quartets and in a small group. Of course some of this will be done as a regular part of his basic music therapy training.

All this time he will be exploring and developing the external part of a musical relationship, responding to rhythmic pulse, melodic phrase and pregnant pause. Not until he starts work in his Intertherapy training in the therapist role will he begin to explore the inner way. (I think it only right to spare one's patients the first faltering steps of a trainee's explorations in responding and feeding back counter-transference emotions).

Even when the trainee has developed dual sensitivity to the inner and outer stimuli, there is still much to be learnt. (This idea of dual sensitivity has an analogy in nature in a certain beetle called a water boatman that can see both above and below the surface of the water as it skims along the pond). The trainee must learn to judge when to respond to a stimulus and when to hold back. For example, a 58 year old woman who was mild and polite in her playing, nevertheless produced a countertransference of violent anger. However, the therapist was only intending to give her a single consultation session and decided that she would not be strong enough to accept or give an airing to this repressed anger of hers in that one session. Therefore he did not react outwardly in passing back this violent emotion.

Working with a schizophrenic man of 32, (the whole case is described in another essay), the patient improvised a very controlled kind of music while imagining finding an old sword in a stream in a forest full of birds and flowers. The countertransference was a feeling of madness which the therapist put into her own music as she thought that the patient could accept a model of a person who could express and yet contain in music these chaotic feelings. In fact this did prove helpful in his longer period of treatment.

The therapist will collect and hoard a store of memories of natural rhythms collected on his walks, so that he has much to draw on in his improvisations. Some years ago a python and grass snake were lodgers in my flat and I was fascinated by the mixture of lightning speed and concentrated torpidity that these creatures showed. It made beautiful movements for improvisation. The experience of all these living rhythms is very healing, counteracting as they do all the dead, mechanical rhythms and vibrations that plague city dwellers.

The musical exchange can bring out a light side of the patient which does not reveal itself in the verbal exchange. A consultant psychotherapist referred a 54-year-old woman to me for therapy. He emphasised that she was a well-educated and articulate lady and I would not have any trouble with her. She had various conversion symptoms from time to time, although at the time of her referral she was not suffering from any one particular symptom. She had mentioned that when she wrote an application form, her handwriting became very jagged and strange, and she did not think that this would make a very good impression on the personnel officer. So for our first improvisation I suggested that we use the title "Application Form." As soon as I switched on the tape recorder she started talking as she played; not talking to me, as she was not even looking in my direction, but talking to herself. Later, when I played back the tape, she talked again with much animation, staring straight at the tape recorder as if she were answering it back. I do not think that the psychotherapist had any idea that there was such a dissociated side of her, from their purely verbal exchange. It was very useful to us to be able to get in touch with it in this way.

Another time I was seeing a middle-aged stockbroker who was suffering from impotence. He seemed a very dull, drab and ordinary man from his speech, indeed he did not seem to have an ounce of poetry in him. But we improvised to an imagination exercise of watching a "Cave Mouth in the Forest" to see what would emerge. His music was delightfully sensitive and delicate and he said that he saw, in his inner eye, a cloud of butterflies emerge from the cave and he followed them into the forest. This delicate sensitivity and imagination was that part of him that was least developed in his everday life. Just as he rejected this side of himself, he then rejected the analytical music therapy that brought it out of him. I never saw him again. Perhaps by now he has retired and is writing poetry on a butterfly farm, perhaps he has married a little Butterfly. But I must curb my imagination and continue with the serious business of the work.

When faced with a patient, the first thing that the therapist must do is to try and find the healing music behind the patient's words. This will lead him to the repressed emotion and the missing potential. Some patients have sufficient insight to be adept at finding just the right verbal title for revealing this emotion, but others will always lead the therapist away from it, and the therapist will have to choose the title himself if any serious work is to be done. Mind you, if you know that you have time to work, it does no harm to ease the situation now and then with a lighter, less ponderous session when you really enjoy playing together in both senses of the word. But sometimes you must grab at the chance to do some important work.

For example: I was working with a 36 year-old manic-depressive patient who had mentioned that she had not had a menstrual period for four and a half months and she feared that she must be having an early menopause. That day she was quite elated and when we came to improvise she wanted to play "Sunshine." However, I thought we had better explore the feelings about the early menopause. She tolerated our music only for a very short while and got in touch with sadness at not having a baby. The very next day she had her period again. The pattern of her illness was to escape from depressive facts by rocketing into her elation, at which time she needed help to get down to the bedrock of the reality that was depressing her and see where she could go from there.

As I mentioned before, the relationship of the therapist to the patient is often that of the "container" to the "contained." The therapist will contain all the extremes of emotion that the patient pours out. This necessitates that he himself has been in contact with the extremes of his own emotion with a good container; otherwise such outbursts might catch him off his guard and overwhelm him.

This is why I continue to state that a trainee analytical music therapist must experience this type of music therapy in the patient position before he launches out into being therapist to another person. The danger is either that he becomes overwhelmed by the strength of his own response to the patient's emotion, or that his suppression of feelings inhibits her expression and what occurs is a kind of pseudo-therapy, very nice, polite and manageable but not getting to the depths of the pain. The patient should never at first, feel exposed and alone with her emotion but, though she may not even consciously hear the therapist's music, she will feel held and enabled to go through the complete cycle of the emotional experience when anger turns to sadness and then to peace. It is for this reason that I prefer to use the piano for most of the time. The greater volume provides a holding matrix for even the loudest drumming and the ability to change the harmony gives one a useful control of mood.

Given an emotionally-freed mother, (and it is not her fault if she isn't one) the normal healthy baby will have learnt to have the complete experience of anger through raging, or sadness through sobbing, or transports of delight with wild gyrations and happy cries turning into peace while safely held in his mother's arms. But not all mothers can take this. Perhaps nobody was able to allow them to do this as children.   Such bodily-expressed emotion does not tear the loved child apart but, because the body gets tired and then relaxes, it offers him a certain fulfillment and satisfaction, a trust in letting his body express what he feels at that early time of innocence and inability to do much harm with it.   Also it is important that he discovers the peace of the bodily relaxation that ensues.   The analytical music therapy improvisation is a symbolic experience of this relationship which is a healing experience in its own right.   It creates a safe playground for the emotions.   It is sad when grown human beings only discover the expression of such feelings through vandalism and inter-personal violence without the possibility of any containment other than prison (an expensive "university of crime"), and no ensuing relaxation and peace for anyone.

The musical relationship offers a quite different kind of working partnership from either the adult working alliance or the transference relationship.   In the latter the patient is working out unfinished business on the therapist as if he was someone else who had been significant in her life.   It can also be a genuine peer relationship of fighting, teasing or mutual caressing in sound.   Or it can be a symbiotic infant-feeding experience.   The patient herself can become the angry parent or withering teacher and reverse the transference roles to see how the therapist likes feeling what she did in the past.   If you, my reader, are a parent or teacher, don't get at me for seeing this at this point from the patient's side.   I am in the process of treating her. I have also sometimes been desperately harrassed by life in this world and have therefore from time to time been an angry mother to three lively sons, and I am sure I was not always a totally inspiring teacher. I probably was not always the perfect patient either.

In this area of musical meeting the therapist cannot be like Freud's cold decisive surgeon or the mirror that gives nothing of itself. In his music the therapist gives of the deepest, richest and most sensitive part of himself.   He is not an accompanist, though sometimes he will play that role to help the patient bring out her expression. Very often he is not playing the role of a separate person in his music but introducing the patient to a lesser-known side of herself.   In the introduction of my book Music Therapy in Action, Dr. E. G. Wooster writes:

These 'mad' parts - and I don't think that these are exclusive to overtly psychotic patients - may be dissociated impulses or perceptions, groundless fears, or bodily symptoms on the one hand or out of touch, rigid defensive structures on the other.

Many patients have found it very comforting, even if painful, to be initiated into a form of musical dialogue with these frightening undeveloped and hitherto unrecognised parts of themselves. After sorting out the confusions and the personality- splits enough to be able to choose the most appropriate form for the musical improvisation, the music therapist himself takes on the role of the patient's warring feelings in their musical dialogue. In the Splitting Technique, the therapist uses the patient's artificial projection to bring the disowned feelings back into the patient's awareness and afterwards they discuss the reactions to this (Priestley, 1975, 12-13).

Very often the patient is quite unaware of the therapist's music while she plays, and only when they hear the playback will she hear the containing, holding music that enabled her to play as she did. Sometimes, astonishingly enough, therapist and patient will play a complicated question-answer phrase pattern but the patient will have had no conscious awareness of doing this at all. It happens by being somehow fused together as a unit at a very deep level.

As an example, a hospitalised young man of 26 was playing some music about not being in control of his life. In the countertransference, the therapist was aware of a pulsing feeling of fear. As he put this into the music, the patient at once picked up the theme on the cymbal and quickly brought the music to a resounding climax. Afterwards he said that he felt relieved as if something oppressive on his head had lifted. He likened the feeling of not being in control of his life to being in his repressive Catholic day school where he used to go to communion in a state of mortal sin rather than have to say 400

Hail Mary's for masturbating. But the point of this example is that he said that he had never heard the therapist's music. He thought that he had made that crescendo on his own initiative and, indeed, as the therapist's pulsing fear music was expressing the feelings from the countertransference, in a way he had.

Quite often important insights and realisations take place when the patient hears the playback, and miraculously, musically-untrained patients will, more often than not, be able to recognise the places in the music where important inner imaginings or feelings were being expressed in their music. Sometimes the therapist will need to emphasise by musical means that he and the patient are two separate persons and offer the patient a musical confrontation. But this cannot be done too soon. It seems that at first in the improvisation the patient is in the same state of consciousness as a happy and contented infant who is a bit vague as to whether the nipple that feeds him and the arms that carry him are also wonderfully satisfying parts of himself.

When the music has been played, together the therapist and patient will discuss their experience and at this time it can be quite interesting for the therapist to observe what, if anything, the patient does with the beaters of the xylophone. A single 37 year old lecturer with obsessional neurosis played some music about various emotions; when he came to "Love" he moved the beaters together in one hand which hinted that he felt ready for a closer rletionship.

A suicidally depressed nurse with a great fear of close relationships, held the beaters in one hand but always had a finger in between them. This could express her distrust of even the closest relationship and her need to control it. This patient brought me many presents and always said that if she could not pay for the therapy she would leave. It marked an important step in her ability to trust when she started re-training on a grant, found herself short of money and was able to accept my invitation to pay me what she could afford until her financial position improved. I noticed that at this time her two beaters were held together with no controlling finger in between. My interpretaions of my patients' holding of the beaters does not indicate that all patients holding the beaters in this way would be having similar feelings. It would be too easy to accept them as universally applicable. The therapist must always be intuitively sensitive to his patient, himself, the situation in the present and the patient's past.

Some patients draw sharp distinctions between the speaking and playing areas in the work room. When they have finished playing they move rapidly back to the speaking area with its two comfortable chairs. It seems that these patients reveal more and stronger feelings in their music than in their words, they then want to disown the feelings and keep their thinking rational and uncontaminated by these disturbing elements. There are no hard and fast rules about interpreting these moves from musicial to verbal areas; however it can be rewarding to the therapist to try and de-code the messages inherent in them so as to get to know more about how the patient feels concerning these two modes of functioning and their relationship to one another.

In the improvisation the therapist offers the patient the opportunity to allow some of the chaos inside her to be expressed. This can be quite a threatening experience. A great part of life is spent in defending ourselves against inner chaos, getting it out of our inner world by externalising it into areas of disorder in our homes, relationships or our opinions of the political party that we do not favour. Therefore it can be reassuring to the patient if the various other elements of the session such as time-keeping, the furniture, the order of the instruments and the times of the sessions all have a reliable feeling of order in their arrangement. For it is the feeling of safe continuity and predictability - a firm rhythm of life - that gives a child, or a patient, the courage to take a step forward, to explore new areas and to grow. She herself needs to be the changing element rather than having to adapt to in-therapy changes.

Although one can often describe the patient's music as being somewhat chaotic, that is not to say that it is without meaning. The choice of instrument, the choice of high or low pitch, the dynamics, the pattern of the melody and the rhythmic or arhythmic pulse, are all consciously or unconsciously determined. Nothing is without meaning.

Sometimes, however, the meaning of the music is not to express the feelings of the player but rather to defend herself against them. For example: a 48 year old hysterical woman with an encapsulated delusional system, played some music about her dream. In this dream her family were all sitting round reading and she talked to them but they did not respond. Suddenly a canary flew into the room and seemed to be going towards the lighted electric fire. She screamed for someone to turn it off, no one did and she just managed to turn it off herself as her husband grabbed her wrists and held her fast. Her music was mild and pleasant in a gentle rhythm. She only played on the xylophone, ignoring the big tom-tom, gong and cymbal. Afterwards she said that she had been seething with anger, she wanted to knock over the family table and really make a scene. She was furious with her husband as he had held her like that in real life. But none of this anger was expressed in music and I knew nothing of it until we talked. In life, too, she usually had a curious symptom in her head when she got into a provoking situation. She talked about her head "pulling up." In fact the one time when she told me that she had let her anger run wild she had been completely uncontrolled and scratched great weals down her husband's arm. One could say that she really lost her head on that occasion. It was not just "pulled up" but now pulled off.

Many times the therapist had tried to get her to express her anger on the drum but the patient always refused. If she could use this emotion in a controlled setting and allow this chaotic area of the psyche to be expressed and shared, she would be well on the way to losing her unpleasant symptom and using her aggression constructively. But the trouble about an encapsulated system is that it is very difficult to access. There was an area of function in her mind like a reverberating circuit, that just went round and round like an unstoppable record.

While improvising, the therapist may be strongly or faintly aware of the patient's hidden feelings through the countertransference as described in the last chapter. For example: a manic-depressive patient playing very angry music produced in the therapist a feeling of deep sadness. The therapist gave this musical expression and the patient's music went very, very quiet and she said later, "When you played that, it was me".

This same response occurred with another manic-depressive patient who was playing about being Unwanted. Her own playing was fragmented and snatchy and when she heard the very calm but sad music that the countertransference produced from the therapist she played very quietly and tried to join in. "I tried to join you as you were playing just what I felt," she said.

Sometimes inner experiences that are not ready to be put into words can be expressed in the music. I had a schizophrenic male patient of 30 who somehow contrived to make the therapeutic session into an ideal nest where no negative emotion was expressed. For a time I went along with this but then I began to express freely in music the countertransference of rage and madness that came up. Later, after a session in which he chose to play "Love," he agreed to explore "Hate" which he experienced as angry then cynical, and lastly a kind of weariness which was the state that he had been in for some time.

Occasionally, when playing with a patient, a noble tune will emerge like a sunrise, embodying feelings of hope and affirmation. When this has happened to me it has reinforced my hope for the successful outcome of the treatment and I have not been disappointed.

For some therapists the expression in music of the counter-transference feelings has a peculiar force while one is improvising. There can be turbulent currents of fear, anger, sadness, rapture and even complicated feelings like the fear of breaking the notes. To the trainee I would give the paradoxical instruction which my teacher of improvisation composer Professor Alfred Nieman gave me: "Hold back and throw yourself in!" He needs to express the feelings but not to be taken over by them. They will threaten to overwhelm him at his weakest point and that is where he must hold back and hang on to himself. The patient will try to split him in two and crucify him but with the music he can hang on to the wholeness. I realise that if the reader has no experience of this work this paragraph will seem nonsensical but when the trainee has had some experience he will know what I mean and I hope my words will be helpful.

The power of music has always been known and used in various ways. I will conclude this chapter with a quotation from the 5,000 year-old "I Ching" (Wilhelm translation, 1951): "Music has power to ease tension within the heart and to loosen the grip of obscure emotions. The enthusiasm of the heart expresses itself involuntarily in a burst of song, in dance and the rhythmic movement of the body...It fell to music to glorify the virtues of heroes and thus to construct a bridge to the world of the unseen" (p. 72). It is up to the trained analytical music therapist to see that this bridge is strong enough for its noble healing purpose.

Essay Fifteen

Some Basic Concepts
Of Freud And Klein

This essay will give a very brief idea of some of the concepts of Sigmund Freud and Melanie Klein (one of his followers whose original contributions are especially important to the work of analytical music therapists). It is hoped that this may act as an appetiser to Freud's forty-two Introductory Lectures on Psychoanalysis (Volumes 15 and 16 of Complete Works), his seven New Introductory Lectures (Volume 22), and Klein's 38 publications possibly preceded by Hannah Segal's book, Klein (1979).

Freud

Freud was born in 1856 (100 years after Mozart), studied medicine in Vienna, with a special interest in neurology, and worked there until 1938, meanwhile marrying, and fathering six children. In 1938, due to the Nazi annexation of Austria, he had to move from Vienna to London where he eventually died in 1939. He first studied hypnosis under Charcot in Paris in 1885 and on returning to Vienna, using this method, he discovered the unconscious process and came upon the idea of free-association (letting the patient speak whatever ideas came to mind however bizarre or debauched) using this instead of hypnosis. The patient lay on a couch and Freud interpreted the material produced (making the unconscious conscious), basing his theories on this material. He called this process psychoanalysis. Through examining his own dreams and parapraxes (slips of the tongue) Freud analysed himself, as far as this is possible, but later stipulated that all future analysts must undergo analysis by a previously analysed analyst before they analyse others.

Freud formulated the then-existing concept of the unconscious (whose contents influence people without their knowledge) in a topographical model of conscious, pre-conscious and unconscious; and also a structural model consisting of super-ego, exerting a moral pressure on the rational; thinking ego; and an id, consisting of sexual and aggressive instincts hungry for gratification. The ego has to juggle with the conflicting demands of the superego, id and reality.

Freud described the unconscious dreamtime mode of mentation as being a primary process with, where necessary, hallucinated wish-fulfillment working according to what he described as the pleasure principle; and a conscious, rational, secondary process of thinking being guided by the reality principle. This allowed the thinker to tolerate considerable frustration on the way to gratification.

We notice primary process thinking in our more disturbed hospital patients; and, to a certain extent, it is used meaningfully by some poets, artists and musicians, for the child self is the root of the artist in mankind.

Another important concept for analytical music therapy, because one has to deal with it over and over again in treatment, is the repetition compulsion. This is a process whereby the patient returns over and over again in dreams and in reality to a point of traumatic fixation hoping desperately but ambivalently for a corrective emotional experience. However, she usually succeeds in setting up her situations so that she re-experiences the original disappointment and can tell the world: "I told you so, this is my fate".

As an example, a patient who was an only child had experienced acute feelings of jealousy and envy of the parental relationship. In later life she was always finding herself in trianglar relationships and frantically hanging on to one or other member of the trio in order not to be in the child's position of being the one left out of the parent's bed. In her case she was repeating the position but desperately preventing the original constellation. In the case of meetings with devoted couples of all kinds, she found that usually the captured member of the triangle gently disengaged himself to bring some parity into the situation which left her feeling once more desolate and rejected, the little one left out. She could not feel as one of three equals; she was either in a one-to-one with the third member left out, or she herself was abandoned. Her awareness of this repetition compulsion was somewhat helped by exploring musically the feelings of being each member of such a triangle: the capturer, the captured and the outsider. However, the feelings about these positions had to be worked through and pointed out repeatedly before she could sustain this awareness and be able and willing to alter her behaviour in a triangle situation.

Freud's theory of psychosexual development was new and startling. He called sexual desire and hunger "libido" and he maintained that it was in existence, in one form or other, from birth. At first people were very shocked at the idea of infant sexuality. Childhood had always been regarded as a time of purity and innocence. Freud wrote that so as not to act against their belief and intentions, people disregard the sexual activities of children, which is quite a feat, or else they scientifically see them in a different light.

At birth a baby's chief interest in life is feeding from the breast, which he does by sucking. As a baby gets older one can see that feeding is a very exciting and wholly satisfying experience. About this Freud wrote that the starting point of the whole of sexual life was sucking at the breast and this was the unequalled prototype for all sexual satisfaction returned to in fantasy later in time of need. The baby's blissful satisfaction and relaxation after a feed is repeated in later life after orgasm, if one is lucky.

The pleasure in feeding is subsequently carried over into the baby's sucking of its lips, tongue and fingers. The mouth and lips are the first erotogenic zones to be explored. This first time of obtaining pleasure and satisfaction through the mouth Freud called the oral phase. As a mother with breast-fed children I must add that there is also a great deal of lively mother-infant relationship during this phase including vocal exchange, stroking and long periods of eye contact. The oral phase is never entirely outgrown, in that many adults hark back to it not only in kissing but sometimes self-destructively through such activities as smoking, over-eating, alcoholism and taking non-prescribed drugs, all of which may provide momentary pleasure and relaxation at the expense of later health.

In analytical music therapy I have often noticed that, after some six to twenty sessions, some of my covertly psychotic patients who had taken overdoses before being referred, gave clear evidence of being in touch with their first oral phase. They looked at me with strange, unfocused, wondering eyes, as if a marvelous memory were about to dawn on them, feeling their lips from side to side with the index finger of their dominant hand. At this time our music has had a blissful, baby quality with many glissandi on the xylophone. While usually lacking the eye contact of the contented mother and baby dyad, our improvisations have had the pleasing mutuality of this time, and even though the patient will say, "I didn't hear your music," these very words indicated an awareness of conflict-free non-awareness. This is the very first meeting place, a rich experience for both parties.

A twenty-seven year-old mother, who had started off the session by weeping because she missed her own dead mother, played music about talking to her mother. The flowing glissandi were followed by a bouncy theme that put me in mind of my own infant sons' delight with themselves and the world after breast feeding. The patient said afterwards that she felt "security." She looked relaxed and glowing.

The second oral phase of cannibalistic sadism is sometimes portrayed by cutting cymbal clashes. Infants also feel pleasure in the free acts of defecation and elimination. Both these areas are connected with loving care from the first-carer which may sometimes, in analysis, be remembered as seduction. It is in this next anal phase that the infant first experiences inhibition from the external world as he makes strenuous efforts at sphincter control in order to please his carer. There is usually a power struggle with regard to the time and place of his "gift" of faeces. This "gift" is the origin of the connection between money and faeces (i.e., "stinking rich," "filthy lucre," and so on). It is a gift from his own inside; a letting go and a relief of tension; a bringing out of his own inner contents and a creative act, possibly later to be symbolised by various artistic productions.

In music therapy the power struggle of the anal phase is usually experienced on the drums, often with quite sadistic fantasies of killing or crushing or breaking in pieces; or it can take an urethral aspect and be flooding, poisoning or overwhelming in rapid music that is prolonged unless it breaks off sharply in fear. It must not be taken that all glissandi indicate that the patient is at the oral stage or all drumming indicates anal phase activity. Just as for an eskimo there are many words for snow, for the music therapist there are many shades of expression in a musical sound.

Later on the child explores other areas of his body, and discovering his genitals, he finds that he can give himself pleasure by masturbation, thus becoming autoerotic. This ushers in the phallic phase, usually between the ages of three and six. Freud said that at this time a boy imagines that everyone---his mother included---has a penis. When he first sees a female in the nude he denies what his eyes see, as the thought that she could have been castrated is so frightening. Freud states that the fetishist continues to disavow the lack of a female penis and substitutes his fetish object for this. Girls, Freud said, become very envious when they see that boys are fitted out with an additional organ with which they can urinate while standing, and they turn against their mothers for not providing them with one.

About this time small children become very attached to the parent of the opposite sex, often stating that they want to marry them. The same-sex parent becomes a hated rival, though sometimes this feeling is disguised as solicitude by a reaction-formation. This is called the Oedipus Complex after the Greek myth in which Oedipus did everything to escape fulfilling the prediction of the Theban oracle that he would kill his father and marry his mother; but nevertheless discovered at last that that was just what he had done unknowingly, and in his anguish he blinded himself. Freud wrote that one of the most notable origins of guilt which tormented neurotics was the Oedipus complex. The fear of castration and of the giant rival parent leads the boy to give up the hope of marrying his mother and to lose his rivalry of his father by identifying with him and working towards the tasks of manhood.

At the same time there can be a negative Oedipus Complex so that the child clings to the same-sex parent and feels the opposite-sex parent as a rival. Herein lies the root of homosexuality. Freud reckoned that the introjection of aspects of the parents presaged the dissolution of the Oedipus Complex. At this time children go through an infantile neurosis developing such symptoms as phobias and obsessions caused by the repression of the sexual and aggressive impulses.

The knowledge of infantile sexuality is essential for the understanding of sexual perversions. Freud wrote that the relinquishment of the reproductive function was a uniting feature of all perversions, and the actual sex life of a child, if any, was thus of necessity of a perverse nature.

So adult perverse sexuality is no more than one part of the

polymorphously perverse infantile sexuality split off and magnified in order to claim its own peculiar satisfactions. This comes about because the libido is what Freud called "fixated" at an earlier level. For normal sexual functioning the individual should have reached the pubertal genital phase in which the young person seeks to find sexual satisfaction with a partner, or through masturbation with a fantasy of a partner. But still the libido can move easily from aim to aim, and normal adult sexuality can satisfy many levels of function, as Hanna Segal (1964) writes,"One organ may be substituted for another and take over its functions. In phantasy, the anus can take the place of the mouth, the penis can replace the breast as an object of oral desires."

Freud described neurosis as the negative of perversion. In other words instead of a perversion being acted out as a source of satisfaction, it can remain in the unconscious (which Freud described as a special area of the mind, closed off from the rest) as a secret desire which nevertheless guiltily draws attention to itself through the medium of a symptom. This may be in any part of the body and disturb any function. The sense of this nonsensical symptom will be contained in the patient's unconscious mind and the psychical work of analysis aims to make conscious what is pathogenically unconscious. However, the knowledge must be given and received in such a way as to bring about an internal change in the patient. Before this can take place a good deal of resistance to this therapy may have to be worked through. Feelings and phantasies long forgotten may need to come to memory, and vital connexions will have to be made between things kept quite separate in the conscious mind of the patient.

As regards the music of the phallic phase, there is not the merging or biting of the oral phase, or the power struggle or grandiose generosity of the anal phase but some sense of identity without, however, much awareness yet of the therapist's music. Genital phase music, on the other hand, is reciprocal; it gives and takes and has awareness of the other and can give a special kind of pleasure to both patient and therapist. But there is no rigid structure between phases, the one can blend into the other in one improvisation so that at one moment the therapist will be a containing, fusing part of the patient and the next minute a chopping block, and then, perhaps, part of a scintillating duet. He must remain very sensitive and flexible but, paradoxically, firm and unyielding too, when necessary.

The theory of defence mechanisms was amplified by Anna Freud and other analysts, and is discussed in another essay herein. These words are written only to open a door to regions with which some students may already be quite familiar and others will surely explore for themselves much more thoroughly later on.

Klein

Melanie Klein was born in Vienna in 1882, the youngest of four children, two of whom died early, leaving her with a tendency to depression and a feeling that it was her duty to develop herself and achieve something in her life.

She married an engineer at twenty-one and had two of her own three children before she started her analysis with Ferenczi. He encouraged her to work with children analytically. She responded to this and developed her own play analysis interpreting the child's play with tiny toys in place of free association. In 1917 she first met Freud and two years later read her first psycho-analytical paper to the Hungarian Society. By 1921 she was also analysing adults. In 1922 her divorce occurred and in 1924 she had a very much valued nine-month analysis with Karl Abraham (who had said "The future of psychoanalysis lies in play technique"). This was terminated by his death, after which Klein conducted a regular and rigorous self-analysis for some years. In 1925 she came to lecture in England and settled there from 1926 till her death in 1960.

It was through her work with children that Klein first began to develop her theories and latterly these enabled patients to be accepted for analysis who would not previously have been thought suitable. These were, for example, borderline (between neurotic and psychotic) patients, delinquents, patients with psychosomatic illnesses and character disorders, the analysis of all of whom requires an understanding of the paranoid-schizoid position and the place of envy.

Klein believed that there is a fragile ego existent from birth imbued with a strong fear of disintegration. She believed that the infant deals with this anxiety by splitting off the good, warm, comforting, gratifying experience of its mother from the painful, hungry, wet, cold lack-of-a-mother experiences. The mother is as yet only a part object (breast) for the baby who is thus aware of an ideal breast into which he has projected his good feelings (or life instinct) and a persecuting breast into which he has projected all his angry, sadistic feelings (or death instinct). (The use of the word "object" here is in the sense of an object of affection rather than an inanimate object).

At this stage of the baby's development Klein believed that there was no consciousness of the lack of the mother as such, but only of pains and discomfort as coming from a persecuting, hating breast. Klein followed Abrahams who delineated a pre-ambivalent oral phase, a second, sadistic, cannibalistic oral phase coinciding with the arrival of teeth, an anal expulsive phase, followed by a second sadistic anal retentive phase.

The experience of the persecuting object, comprising a retaliation for the infant's biting, cannabalistic desires, is often of many sadistic, chewed-up, persecuting objects in contrast to the single ideal breast.   This position Klein called the paranoid-schizoid position: "paranoid" because the infant experiences the persecutory anxiety of his projected hate and sadism, and "schizoid" because he makes the split between the good and the bad experiences.

The fact that this is a position rather than a phase explains it as a certain way of interpreting reality which is not necessarily chronological. A great many adults are going about their daily round regarding life from this position, either permanently or just temporarily due to regression caused by stress. A therapist might congratulate himself on being the patient's "ideal object" while all the other hospital staff are regarded as persecutory, attacking objects, if he did not realise that it would only take a snap of the fingers to reverse the projections; and that until he can become the container for both kinds of feeling he will not be able to help the patient very much. Such a positive transference can be extremely seductive to the therapist who could be led into all kinds of excesses; but a good astringent relationship with colleagues plus a warm and loving relationship elsewhere can be useful prophylactics.

One of my patients, a middle-aged woman, subject to depressions, saw herself as a black blob over a long period of treatment; then, when improvising about a new room to which she was moving, she brought the ideal image of herself as a jewel set in madonna-blue velvet. In the next session we split these two images between us, alternately being the ideal and bad objects. Tremendous banging on the drum expressed her black blob loneliness and anger,it completely blotted out my jewel music. Then reluctantly, as she played being the jewel, she experienced my black blob music as being a child in a tantrum who needed to be loved. It was a very nice rehearsal of the merging of these two objects with the healing ascendance of the loving feelings, and an either/or approach to herself becoming a both/and.

Ferenczi did not work with Klein's negative transference and the realisation of this lack may have helped her in the construction of these theories.

The next position described by Klein was the "depressive position" which might normally develop at a time when the infant is three to six months old. At this time the infant becomes aware of his mother as a whole object, able to remove herself from his presence, or to return of her own volition rather than be controlled by his hallucinatory fantasies. There is sadness at the loss of the mother when she absents herself or cannot be seen. There is also toleration of the conflict that his ambivalent feelings towards her bring. By this time the infant should have introjected a whole mother, a whole father and a creative parental couple. Defence against this last may consist of a hated/hating stuck-together mother-father imago which is the basis for many two-headed, four-legged nightmare images, the envious destructive hate towards the couple's intercourse being reflected back by this persecutory monster.

When patients develop into the depressive position they will suddenly begin to show concern for the therapist. A nurse patient brought me professional articles on the need for sleep when she thought that I looked tired, this was at a time when her ambivalence (which one could hear in our music) was particularly strong, and her own sleep pattern was actually quite disturbed.

Klein dated the working through of the Oedipus Complex as during the time of the achievement of the depressive position but said that the first parental introjects are part objects i.e. breasts and penises rather than whole objects. It was this rudimentary, harsh, sadistic super-ego that Klein analysed in her small patients. In 1977, she wrote "it became clear to me that the super-ego, as conceived by him (Freud), is the end product of a development which extends over years." This primitive super-ego behaved by talion law (an eye for an eye) with all the creative sadism of the child's fantasies towards his parents.

Klein discovered that many children fantasised scooping out the insides of the mother's body to steal milk, faeces, father's penis, and babies and then developed a terror of their own bodies being attacked.

I treated a patient who had lived on a houseboat for five years, lovingly building it and painting it every spare moment of his life. He lived rather a solitary life and had difficulties in interpersonal relationships, especially with girls. When he began therapy with me, he consistently came to his session half an hour to twenty minutes late. My theory was that he was making reparation to this boat/mother for attacking her insides and that this attack was symbolised in the present by his attacks on our session time. I interpreted that he was robbing and attacking my session and his guilt and consternation were striking. Next time he came on the dot of nine.

At this time, with the awareness of love as well as hate toward their objects, children will try to make reparation. They also develop the capacity to use symbolism so that, for example, cleaning out the nursery drawers and mending the toys could be a reparation for a fantasy for exploring and robbing the mother's insides.

Any hindrance to this process of symbol formation and free fantasy will be seen in the inhibition of the child's play and epistemophilic instinct, as Klein, in her early work, described it. It means, of course, love of knowledge. Regarding this process, Dr. E. G. Wooster of London wrote (1986): "This potential sexual energy of the young child expressing itself in curiosity, pleasure in exploring, of fondling and handling, of role-playing towards identification, including swapping of boy and girl roles, has its beginnings, of course, in early life in the home and is vulnerable all along the road to development to the point of school where anatomical curiosity can pass into science, curiosity about our origins can pass into history, of exploring by geography, of fondling and handling by art and woodwork, of role-playing imaginatively through literature, of pleasure in identity swapping through foreign languages, of pleasure in the very discovery of symbolism through mathematics and the mechanics of language. "

Klein found that one child felt extremely guilty and unable to learn because for her the schoolhouse symbolised her mother's body, and the teacher symbolised father's penis. When these unconscious phantasies came to light the child's symptoms receded.

This is the time of sublimation; reparation and a manageable amount of envy produce fruitful progress both in the child and in the patients whose loving impulses are not overcome by destructive ones. It is the time of new interests, connected with new symbols, and new aspirations connected with new identifications. Failure of the loving impulses to master the destructive ones, is a primary cause of mental illness when these are directed towards the ego, or psychopathy when directed towards society.

There is also manic reparation, much used by do-gooders and empire-builders, in which the object does indeed receive good things but is kept as a de-valued recipient of this reparative action, on a permanent poor relation, second-class citizen basis, to boost the giver's ego.

The pathway to the depressive position is not always straightforward. In this position there is pain, pining for the good object and guilt at having damaged it. Against all this there are manic defences: denial of love and need for the object, or denial of ambivalence, contempt for the object and phantasies of omnipotent control and trumph over it.

A patient who was shortly to leave therapy, took to reading psychoanalytic books and triumphing over her therapist with her self -interpretations. At the same time she treated the therapist contemptuously as a stupid child. When this was interpreted she worked hard with her feelings of loss of the therapist as a valued object and of the loss of the care by her dead mother, which she experienced as unloving, and of her fury at the pair of them for leaving her.

The depressive position is the fixation point for manic-depressive or depressive illness in that the patient fails to achieve the feeling of having a good internal object. In depression the patient mourns the loss of the object, heaps reproaches on herself and feels utterly devalued and useless. Mourning, which is the loss of a good external object, can trigger off feelings belonging to the depressive position. There can be true mourning followed by a time of enrich-ment and new interests, or the manic defences described above can come into play and the original failure to come to grips with depressive feelings can lead to abnormal mourning or mental illness.

A widow was working through the first year of her mourning well, but her good internal object did not sit securely inside, as she said,"I cannot recall his voice at all." She had somehow severed this link with her husband and felt that even in memory she was cut off from him.

Klein was the first analyst to describe the mechanism of projective identification. There is also an example of this in the essay on ego defences. As another example one can think of a baby so hungry that he thinks he will die, who projects this feeling into his mother. The sensitive mother will realise on the one hand how anxious he feels, yet be able calmly to feed him in a comforting way; thus returning to him the sense that this feeling was manageable. An agitated mother with too many other internal or external problems of her own, might refuse to entertain the projection and make him wait until a time that was convenient to her (by which time his persecutory fears might be well-nigh overwhelming); or she might identify with the projective identification and become as desperate as the baby, possibly damaging him in the process.

If there is the projection of bad parts of the self, the object of these projections is felt to be persecutory. If there is the projection of good parts, then the individual feels that she is depleted, she tends to idealise the object and has a need to control it lest she lose her treasures.

A suicidal wife and mother in her forties, went through a period of idealising me, and then felt it necessary to ring me up after the session to see that I was not thinking things that she did not want me to think.

All this sounds rather esoteric until one has become the target for someone's projective identification then suddenly one understands what Klein was describing in her technical language. Projective identification is a primitive method of communication. It has a strange invasive quality which makes it, at first, very difficult for the object to avoid identifying himself with the projected part or feeling. Personally, I believe that the higher animals are capable of it. I feel also that we are here in the region of the spells and bewitchment of former times.

Narcissistic object relations are based on projective identification. Having projected his good parts into a partner resembling himself in some way, a person idealises his object and has a need to control it, together with a great fear of being enslaved by it. This is the basis of the schizoid fear of loving. Having projected his bad parts into an object, he then fears retaliation and cannot introject the object whom he fears will imprison and control him.

If the therapist cannot work through the negative transference of a patient, the patient then cannot withdraw her bad projection and introject a good-enough therapist object. Thus she may feel forced to terminate the therapy without having the strong, inner dialogue which would help her to make a successful future on her own.

Weakened by excessive splitting and projection, the individual in the paranoid-schizoid position may not have enough ego left to face the depressive position's emotional pain.

Klein's last work was on the importance of envy and gratitude. As the real relationship of the parents, as two separate people, is perceived in the depressive position, the child can experience envy (of one) and jealousy (between three). Sometimes, in phantasy, the parental couple is split up into a good, non-sexual couple and a bad, copulating couple; or the couple is seen, as before described, as a combined parental figure incapable of intercourse as they are permanently united. The object of envy can be spoiled in phantasy or in reality by a child to make it less enviable. For example, a small girl was found poking her finger into her baby brother's eye to render him less attractive to their mother (external destruction); at the same time her older sister said he was anyway an ugly little boy (internal destruction). If there is less, and more manageable envy, that is to say that the envied state or thing is possibly attainable by the envier, then it can be a spur to advancement.

A single patient of mine spent the weekend with an engaged couple - a situation which might produce keen envy - but he solved the problem by coming back radiant. He had, in imagination, stolen all their delightful home-making ideas in readiness for the creation of his own kitchen when he left the hostel where he was rehabiltating.

Klein describes the boy's envy of his mother's body with his father's penis in it, and the girl's envy of her father's penis that makes reparative intercourse with her mother. Envy of the feeding breast can give way to gratitude and later symbolic or real rivalry and emulation. Or the feeling of envy may be so severe that the envying part of the personality is split off, thus exluding a valuable dynamic part of the person. The envy may also destroy the feeding or therapy experience completely.

In one analysis Klein's patient's envying part was felt, terrifyingly, to be madness; but she managed to help the patient to integrate it enrichingly into her personality.

Close to envy comes greed, which makes a person aim at having all the good things for herself, regardless of his own need or the willingness of the other to give. Greedy people are not worried about being envied, anything rather than the pain of being envious. Other people fear very much being envied, their own envy is so destructive; primitive and unconscious that this emotion is feared and avoided in others even at the expense of their own comfort and progress.

A writer's son envied his mother's successful life and productions so much that each time his own first two books were published he suffered a breakdown, being wholly unable to tolerate the stress of enviableness.

As a concluding note, I have not in this essay described the theories of Carl Jung. This is not at all because they are not relevant to analytical music therapy. I believe them to be both relevant and useful to any person trained in analytical psychology. But in spite of the fact that I have now had eleven years of analytical supervision of my work with a distinguished Jungian training analyst, Dr. J. W. T. Redfearn, I felt that my own training and experience in this method has not been extensive enough for me to apply these theories widely in my work. To have had personal work on oneself in a certain method gives one a much deeper understanding of it than mere knowledge gleaned from books, lectures and papers. And I believe that this deeper understanding is necessary if one wants to impart it in any thorough-going way to others with any degree of success.

Essay Sixteen

Defence Mechanisms
And Some Examples

Ego defences are part and parcel of one's psychic life. They help to keep at bay some of the overwhelming anxiety that would otherwise be caused by the awareness of certain threatening feelings, thoughts, impulses and memories. They also help to master and canalise inner forces which might disrupt the function of the ego. In use, they could be likened to the stops on an organ which divert the outgoing air to create certain sounds and not others.

In the animal world different creatures have evolved their own particular defences. Some have surface protections, such as exoskeletons, spines, shells, armour or scales; others take defensive actions, such as death-feigning, rolling up, warning calls and signs, casting tails, flocking, camouflage and burrowing; others use mimicry of weapons such as horns, teeth and claws, or flash colouration. The human ego endeavours to protect itself also in various ways from danger within and without. Love of life, and therefore anxiety about survival, is at the root of all this invention.

In 1926 Freud differentiated two types of human anxiety: traumatic anxiety, in which the ego is overwhelmed by stimuli; and signal anxiety, a more mature response, in which the ego is alerted to danger from either outside or from the super-ego or id. If signal anxiety is experienced, steps can be taken to protect oneself from external danger, and if there is fear of the breakthrough of what the individual fears will be uncontrollable sexual or aggressive instincts, or super-ego attacks, then the defence mechanisms come into action.

The use of a certain amount of ego defences is a normal and necessary part of psychic development. For example, denial and the projection of feelings that one is not yet able to accept as one's own, allows one to observe them in others, and later to recognise and come to terms with them in oneself. Identification with admired objects (people) can help one to develop oneself in imitation of them and grow; introjection of such objects enables one eventually to leave their physical presence without feeling too bereft. Sublimation enables one to use some of the energy of the vital sexual and aggressive drives in a civilised, modified but nevertheless dynamic manner. Examples are: playing a musical instrument instead of indulging in sex indiscriminately, or playing games or sports instead of killing people. But, as in the animal world, too much energy put into defences weakens the person in other ways. Two examples are the dinosaurs who were said by some to have died out because of developing their size at the expense of their brains; or two fighting stags who get their antlers interlocked and starve to death because they cannot then eat.

Human beings who habitually use too many or too bizarre ego defences, have very little freely-circulating energy left to spend on the rest of their life-activities. They become emotionally crippled, devitalised people, sometimes colloquially described as "seized-up rigid," "high-entropy" or "low-energy" types. For example: a boy who projected all his aggression into the environment, felt extremely paranoid and could not take any interest in the outside world at all as he felt it to be so persecutory.

The analytical music therapist works to facilitate a somewhat freer energy flow. The patient's musical expression, in the containing therapeutic dyad, seems to diminish some of the original anxiety about the emotion or memory which was defended against. This allows at least a manageable part of it into consciousness. Some of the super-ego condemnation seems to turn into approval of this socially acceptable emotional outlet, partly because the patient's super-ego can be projected on to the therapist who will prove milder than the patient's own. The patient with faltering ego strength, has this slowly built up through the creation of musical and later verbal structures to hold and work with the threatening emotion.

An emotion given outward expression in the holding presence of a good therapist, does not threaten the ego in the way that does a strong emotion for which no consciously-directed outlet can be found. The latter can find a destructive or personally disruptive outlet by intefering with unconsciously-directed bodily or mental function through incapacitating ego defences or psychosomatic illness. But in this work the therapist will need to proceed very sensitively, respecting the patient's initial need for her defences as they will not have not grown up without good reason.

When improvising with the therapist, sometimes the patient's music expresses her feelings and sometimes, with vehement force, it expresses the strength of one of her defences. It is astonishing to hear a defence, which in verbal exchange seems to be like static armour, turn into a powerful audible dynamic energy through music. Sometimes intense emotion may be expressed in a patient's music but the verbalisation of this emotion may be blocked, and it is especially in such cases that a knowledge of the ego defences can be useful.

The following are some of the fairly common ego defences with, where available, examples from my analytical music therapy (AMT) practice.

REPRESSION renders a threatening impulse or idea unconscious. A patient who had suffered a sexual trauma in her teens had had no experience of sexual desire for twenty-five years until, after five years of AMT, this feeling emerged quite strongly and she felt able to discuss it with her therapist. This was a gentle, gradual process, and not the less manageable and less safe sudden and explosive cathartic breaking through of repressed feelings.

SUBLIMATION is the healthy, alternative conscious channelling of instinctual energies of sex or aggression. Every worthwhile performing musician uses plenty of these equally-balanced sublimated energies. Pupils sometimes lack the de-aggressivised energy which will render their playing soft, flabby and undisciplined at first. However, teachers will occasionally see pupils with iron discipline but no trace of de-sexualised tender or passionate feelings in their playing. An autistic patient who came to see me, at first for violin lessons for two years, was one such case. His rhythm and intonation were faultless but the music was completely lacking in emotional content. A person cannot sublimate drives of which he is totally unconscious. However, during the course of therapy, the patient's freed id energies may find their way into new interests and creative pursuits which have symbolic significance for him.

DENIAL may be the disavowal of some aspect of one's own personality, in which case it operates together with splitting and projection. It may also be the denial of an unwelcome impulse or some painful past experience. In manic-depressive illness, in the manic phase, depression is denied and split off in time into the depressive phase. During the depressive phase the patient can have dreams of being above the ground flying or in a radiant state of happiness which disappears promptly on waking. A patient in his first AMT session took great trouble in pointing out that there was no trace of envy and jealousy between himself and his more successful brother: "We have always been the best of friends." Working with music to the title "Mother," he came upon the memory of the two boys sitting on either side of their father, who was earnestly endeavouring to keep the peace between them. His need for the denial was diminished by the reduction of anxiety through giving his emotion some expression in his music.

SPLITTING can be understood in several ways. First there is the splitting of the self and the identification of the subject with only one part, such as the "good" part in the previous example. Then there is the splitting into several parts and identification with each one in turn as in the hysterically-dissociated character in the film "The Three Faces of Eve." She was alternately inadequate, bad, and later responsible and mature. A certain benign splitting occurs in the helpful observing self-awareness of a person undergoing analytical work or under certain religious and esoteric disciplines at one stage of development. A different kind of splitting is the splitting of objects into good (ideal) and bad (persecutory) because the ambivalence of feeling love and hate for the same person is felt to be too threatening. A great many hospital patients enjoy the rich opportunities for splitting between their therapists, thus the art therapist may be "in" and the music therapist "out" or vica versa. It is vital that the staff concerned meet regularly and repair these splits, rather than act them out for the patient. Denial, splitting and projection form a working trio which impoverishes the ego but may nevertheless serve to keep it intact until a better functioning mode can be evolved.

PROJECTION is the logical consequence of denial. The aspects thus denied are projected and understood as belonging to someone or something outside oneself. For example, a woman patient who had just discovered a very weak, insecure core of herself, denied and projected her strong, capable part on to the hospital staff in general and me in particular. "If only someone would give me a little push," she said. In music we improvised playing alternately the role of this someone-who-pushes and her weak part that needed it. In this way she regained the feeling of her strength and capability. However, her next move was to use it to manipulate her various therapists into taking care of her as the weak self, rather than to use her strength to take care of this newly acknowledged weak self and to give herself the needed little push. But at least it was a movement that could eventually develop into something stronger outside therapy.

INTROJECTION besides being a defence, is one of the normal processes of development. Children introject their images of their parents, in both good and bad aspects, which combine to become their super-egos. This inner mental representation of an external object, enables the client to leave her therapist or the pupil her teacher, and become more self-reliant. As a defence it reduces separation anxiety.

A patient who improvised in the role of her therapist, reproduced what she felt were the therapist's powerful and soothing rhythms in her own music. She felt that the therapist found her difficult to cope with and was to an extent impotent in the face of her helpless dependency. Another ex-patient, now in a helping role, felt that she could only deal with some clients from her introjected "Inner Therapist" or in other words through introjective identification. Introjection is one of the mechanisms of depressives who always see the other person's point of view and agree with it on the principle "If you gobble something up it's done with." Thus they avoid having to use their aggression which they fear has destroyed an introjected object for which they mourn and reproach themselves.

SUPPRESSION is the process of inhibiting a thought or deed by an act of will. The husband of a couple, who my colleague Marjorie Wardle and I saw for some joint sessions, suppressed his anger in the verbal exchange, relying on his wife to express it for him, which she did periodically in a violent uncontrollable manner. However, it did find expression in his drum-beating now and then, and he looked very much better for it with notable relaxation of the jaw muscles, shoulders and hands.

REGRESSION is a move backwards in time, to operating at a more primitive state of development. In a toilet-trained child, for example, it could mean bed-wetting or abandonment of speech as a reaction to a baby sibling coming into the family. Even adults sometimes revert to little helpless gestures when they want to be passively looked after for a fleeting regressive moment.

As a more persistent defence against major anxiety, however, this is not a very reassuring mechanism because there are also hierarchies of anxiety, regressing from the adult's fear of loss of self-esteem, to the adolescent fear of castration, to the younger child's fear of the loss of parental love and approval, to the small child's terror of separation and abandonment.

Freud's oral, anal and phallic phases may describe the points at which a person may be fixated but, in fact, all these different ways of operating and experiencing life are there all the time, like notes on a piano which may be played as required. Patients entering psychiatric hospitals are often quite regressed and also very exhausted from fear and lack of sleep, and sensitive helpers instinctively treat them a little more tenderly at first, though they are never, in my experience, allowed the physical rest they need. However, such sensitive helpers also know when to let go and let them regain their adulthood, which may occur surprisingly quickly.

In order to profit from AMT or any kind of psychotherapy, a certain amount of regression, in the form of agreeing to be the patient and depending on and trusting the therapist, is necessary. That is why we can sometimes come across difficulties in treating our colleagues or anyone who works in a "caring" role. Some of them insist on only being the one in charge because they find the dependent situation very threatening. See the essay entitled "Inner Child."

REACTION-FORMATION is an obsessional defence in which the person behaves in the opposite way to their unconscious infantile impulse which, however, remains unaltered. For example, a patient had always been praised as a faultlessly devoted little mother to the sister who was born when she was seven and of whom she had been unconsciously violently jealous. The unmasking of this emotion was extremely painful to her but it persistently revealed itself in a mother transference as when she left her sessions she would always glance down the passage to the waiting area to see what "new baby" was waiting for my attention.

Reaction-formation can serve a useful purpose in that, for example, the cleanliness of the operating theatre could be thanks to a reaction-formation against coprophilia (pleasure in eating and handling faeces), or a life of devoted service a reaction-formation against the infantile wish to be cruel and sadistic. But it can also be sadly crippling to the person using it and to those around her, and a great strain on the energy flow of the individual concerned.

ISOLATION is another defence, used mostly by obsessional neurotics. The patient manages to isolate certain happenings or a certain happening from his emotions or associations. It is sometimes recognised by a silence accompanied by a certain facial expression or small gesture when a certain subject is mentioned. A sensitive child can recognise, accept and have a life-long fear of this marked-off taboo area in a parent so that she is unable not only to think rationally and constructively in that taboo area herself but any area connected to the original taboo may be affected.

UNDOING is a quasi-magical act undertaken in order to cancel out a previous deed or thought. For example, a patient was compelled to indulge in excessive hand-washing if she even touched any kind of rubbish container; and this was an undoing of anal-sadistic impulses. In another patient such handwashing might endeavour to undo sexual or aggressive impulses, as with Lady Macbeth with her "Out, out, damned spot." Music therapists should be wary of being pushed into performing magical musical undoing through their patients' improvisation titles. They might work in some cases but they would not offer the patient the healing bricks of understanding.

INTELLECTUALISATION is taking everything from an intellectual point of view and thus escaping from any emotional depth or pain. The music cuts through this quite successfully in providing a genuine emotional experience. The problem then is to bring this back into verbalisation. One patient used this defence to look at situations only from the point of view of financial loss or gain. For example, when his girl friend left him he remarked only that this would be cheaper and he could increase his savings.

RATIONALISATION is a way of hiding one's true motivation by finding factual reasons and justification for one's conduct. For example, a patient with a wealth of unconscious aggression, aimed at the therapist in the present but at the patient's father in the past, had a long series of water-tight reasons why she was repeatedly late for her sessions: bus strikes, phone call as she left home, meter-reader called, lost her umbrella, cat vomited on carpet and so on.

PHOBIC AVOIDANCE is a defence in which the individual avoids objects or situations which have become a symbol of that which triggers off her anxiety. For example, a cat jumped into the bedroom of a bridal pair at a critical moment of their wedding night and from then on the wife was frigid and cat-phobic. The cat symbolised the conflict between animal (physical) pleasure and super-ego disapproval. Improvisation can be helpful in getting behind the symbol to the source and feeling of the original anxiety.

COUNTERPHOBIC ACTIVITY is a manic defence. The individual using this takes delight in all such occupations that would terrify a normal person, and experiences triumphant and omnipotent feelings when he survives, and also when he relates these exploits to normally fearful others.

PROJECTIVE IDENTIFICATION is a defence mechanism described by Melanie Klein, in which impulses or, in phantasy, parts of the individual's body, are projected into her objects so that if these are good parts, she feels devalued, dependent on the object and needing to control it, and if they are bad parts she feels persecuted by the object. Through the sense of being persecuted following attacks on her mother's body by projective identification, the child can build up a punitive super-ego even though its mother, in reality, is a kind and loving person.

A young man put into me the feeling that he must be treated as the cherished youngest son. I was aware of this and tried to hand it back to him as a reasonable plea to be treated fairly, but time and time again I found myself falling into the trap of stepping out of the therapist role for a second to spoil him with an answer to an intrusive question or an extra minute after it was time, only to pull myself up to ask myself "What am I doing?".

Sometimes a whole therapeutic team will fall in with a patient's need-of-special treatment, identifying with the projective identification. This defence is a very powerful and primitive way of communicating, it requires real strength and clarity on the part of the therapist meeting it. Reading about it as a concept, I found it quite impossibly hard to take in, but as soon as what was happening in my session was pointed out as being given this name, it made sense as a distinctive interpersonal happening. Narcissistic object relationships (friends who choose friends like themselves) are based on projective identification.

CONFUSION is a defence in which the subject feels himself to be in a disorienting, defensive fog and all attempts to clarify matters end in worse confusion. Various patients have reserved this defence for dealing with either time or money matters. This is not to be confused with psychotic confusion, for example where a manic patient governed by primary process (unconscious) thinking, loses time awareness, or a schizophrenic patient loses the sense of her identity.

DEPERSONALISATION produces a feeling of unrealness of the subject. A neurotic patient, as a child, left her family in the car to buy an ice cream. When she got back the car had disappeared and she experienced this frightening feeling of being unreal. Improvising on this, of course she sounded very real and very anxious.

DEREALISATION produces the feeling that the external world is unreal. Freud had this experience momentarily when he visited the Acropolis which his father had longed to see but had never been granted this wish. The thought of thus going beyond what his father had achieved evoked anxiety which produce this defence. (See Volume 22 of the Complete Works, p. 244).

CONVERSION is the defence in which emotion, either attached or unattached to ideas, is expressed through the medium of physical symptoms. I have sometimes witnessed dramatic "cures" when a patient has played the music of her headache and it has vanished after the improvisation. During my Intertherapy I even lost my own headache while being therapist to my colleague who was playing with tremendous aggression! Many conversion symptoms will convert back into music and thus emotion, but it requires patient work by therapist, patient and her environment before the patient learns to keep the normal channels for emotional expression permanently open. Here the assistance of certain body-work therapies or Eastern body-mind meditation exercises can be very useful.

PSYCHOSOMATIC STATES differ from the defence of conversion in that they are recognisable illnesses. For example, peptic ulcers, psoriasis, ulcerative colitis or bronchial asthma are a few disorders which can be brought on or exacerbated by emotional causes. Music therapists are now widely accepted in clinics for psychosomatic illness in some European countries. I have given AMT sessions to several colleagues now working in such places in Germany.

DISPLACEMENT OF AFFECT occurs when feelings about one person, or thing, are transferred to another, as they also are in the symbols contained in dreams. In Music Therapy in Action (Priestley, 1975), I wrote about a young mother who felt inexplicably angry with her little second daughter because she resembled physically, the young mother's sister who had been found in bed with the child's father. Through musical exploration of the mother's tremendous rage which was not expressed at the time, the emotion was transferred back to the offending sister psychically and withdrawn from the child, who then had a period of loving reocnciliation with her mother in the hospital.

TURNING AGAINST THE SELF occurs when a person uses his aggression or sadism against himself (not necessarily physically). Through violence on percussive instruments patients have been able to turn their aggression outwards again, and after a period of uncertain use (breaking the odd plate or window and having outbursts of anger), they have retrained a measure of controllable de-aggressivised energy to put to good use through healthy self-assertion.

IDENTIFICATION WITH THE AGGRESSOR is a defence in which the patient thinks, "If you can't beat 'em, join 'em." This explains why parents who batter their children produce children who, when they grow up, are inclined to batter their own children in turn. A hospital out-patient who had been battered as a child always asked her husband to come in to the bathroom with her when she bathed her new baby. She was so terrified of identifying with her own battering mother.

REVERSAL is a defence in which there is an about-turn in impulses, thus a man may relate homosexually to defend himself against Don Juan aspirations; sadism may change to masochism and exhibitionism to voyeurism; a person may develop agorophobia to cover a desire for promiscuous conquests; ascetism in adolescents and others may defend against a desire for wild debauchery. Patients have found it helpful to express one side of such reversals in their music while the therapist plays the opposite role and then change roles. This can give them the feeling of the reality of the impulse that is being defended against deep inside them, so they can discuss it with less anxiety and more experience of it in the present.

IDENTIFICATION. Projective identification has been discussed earlier, that leaves us with primary identification which is the state of mind of a baby before it is clearly aware of itself in distinction to others, and secondary identification which is a defence in which the subject identifies with (feels and tries to act like) another person whom he realises is a separate entity. Young children working through the Oedipus complex and desiring to possess the opposite-sex parent, are normally deterred by castration anxiety and driven to identify with the same-sex parent. If this does not happen they can become cross-identified and later feel and relate homosexually temporarily or permanently. A twenty-year-old girl totally changed her taste in music from Spanish to Greek to Italian to Japanese in identification with current boyfriends.

TRIUMPH AND CONTEMPT like denial, are manic defences against feelings of anxiety, depression and/or guilt. They are not only used by patients with manic-depressive illness. A patient whose husband had had a wild affair with the neighbour's foreign cook, treated him with the deepest contempt for twenty years, refusing him intercourse and verbally doing what she called "de-bagging" him in front of others. In this way she successfully hid from herself the deep sadness that his disloyalty had caused her.

PSYCHIC NUMBING can take place in traumatic situations. There is a gentle, protective blunting of feelings which, however, can be recalled cathartically at a later date.

FANTASISING can protect people from the sobering facts of their existence. For example, fantasies of secret and special relationships, like the patient who danced with the Virgin Mary; or of rich and powerful ancestors (adopted or simply maladjusted children sometimes have these); or of omnipotent thoughts and wishes which will transform the world. Fantasies become part of shared human life when sold as films, plays, novels and operas, or when they form part of the mythology or religious stories of any organised group. Phantasies spelled with Ph are those that are unconscious and can be revealed in analysis or other therapies with a consequent gain in energy.

DETACHMENT AND SULKING are forms of withdrawal of interest which are defences against anger, much used by children who feel that the expression of anger could cause loss of love; or those who have not the energy to express their anger openly. It is protective, of course, as totally uncontrolled anger expressed physically is often catastrophic to the point of murder in close relationships.

HUMOUR is a defence against anxiety, anger and depression, which is very much part of normal British life and often used in conjunction with fantasies. In a recent interdisciplinary hospital group where the chaplain was talking of dying and death, the art and music therapists started to laugh uproariously until they had rid their psyches of accretions of stimuli whereupon they admitted the fears that lay beneath their laughter and settled down to share some of them. The relaxing factor of laughter, like improvising music with its gentle physical release of tension, can sometimes enable the person to face the unfaceable after its expression.

When we talk about "getting to know what makes someone tick," a large part of this is learning how to relate to the other person and get the best out of him in spite of his defence mechanisms, or even to profit by them.

Besides the individual defence mechanisms there are character defences. For example, an individual's personality can be basically phobic, hysterical, obsessional, schizoid, hystrionic, hypomanic or it can approach the world through a false self. Generally speaking I have found that the music of the obsessional patient sounds a bit stunted, the hypomanic's compulsive, the schizoid's without dynamism, the hystrionic will not stop, the phobic's can sound rapid and anxious, the hysteric's is dynamic and dramatic, and the music of the character with the false self, if she is playing from her uncultivated real part, sounds chaotic, varied and undisciplined; but there are, of course always exceptions.

Anything can be used as a defence: religion, art appreciation, gardening, psychoanalysis, ornithology are only a few examples. But, like fantasy and humour, such defences can sometimes also be used constructively and creatively to enrich a healthy life or community.

Essay Seventeen

Music, Freud And
The Port Of Entry

In the collected works of Freud there are only six references to music as opposed to forty-two references to art. I will use one of the former to look at the different ways in which music is used in analytical music therapy dyadic improvisations.

In Freud's "The Dream-Work" (1900) he writes that if, as happens in Don Giovanni, he hears a little music and someone says that it is out of Mozart's Figaro, several memories are aroused in him all at once, none of which were able to enter his consciousness by themselves (See Volume 5 of Complete Works, p. 497). Freud regards this first-heard phrase as a "port of entry" which puts the network into a state of excitation. This, he thinks, may also be the case with unconscious thinking.

For Freud, music opens a door to excitations accompanied by a number of different recollections. In music therapy we can discern three distinct mental operations as such "ports of entry."

The first operation is free emotional musical expression varying in pitch and rhythm according to the player's moods. The rhythm may or may not have a recognisable pulse but I have never heard it turn into a compulsive heavy beat. This operation in turn divides into three different expressive happenings.

The first, which I will call 1a, occurs when the emotion is expressed musically and is able to be acknowledged with the intellect, allowing a stream of accompanying memories and thoughts to arise in the mind.

The second, 1b, allows musical expression but is followed by a block in thinking. I call this experience the "resistance vacuum." A resistance vacuum is the psychic space which would otherwise be occupied by a link between emotion and thought. Bion (1955) wrote: "In this state of mind emotion is hated; it is felt to be too powerful to be contained by the immature psyche; it is felt to link objects and give reality to objects which are not-self and therefore inimical to primary narcissm" (p. 308).

In this vacuum, there is a resistance to linking the emotion which is so clearly expressed in the music, to thought. Strangely enough, when the player tries to think following the musical expression, the energy of the resistance is not experienced but only a curiously baffling unattached emptiness.

In the third, 1c, the resistance vacuum is covered up by a strong aural impression of the music. This is a more sophisticated defence against acknowledging the emotion, in that it can be limited to thought, but only regarding the musical content and the impression of the sounds, and not the emotion.

The second operation is the musical expression of the resistance vacuum itself. It is usually a monotonous kind of ostinato. It seldom ranges over more than a few tones and is reminiscent of the repeated chants of some of the more ancient religions for examples Zoroastrian Fire Temple chants and the chants of Thai Buddhists. This, however, can lead to the release of memories, thoughts amd feelings.

The third operation is the actual musical expression of the resistance energy which is blocking out the painful emotion that the resistance vacuum is covering. This music is a compulsive beating which is unpleasant to listen to. This, again, is usually followed by the baffling, empty experience of the resistance vacuum. However, occasionally some of the underlying emotion can be contacted. It puts one in mind of the auto-destructive rhythmic head-banging of some autistic children. One also wonders whether some of the heavy beat music, disliked so much when it comes through the wall at 3 AM, satisfies Operation 3 in others at second hand. In this way the listener-for-pleasure, can resonate to a kind of sullen rage without actually being in a position to know what the painful emotion behind it is about, and therefore can be caught in a mindless vicious circle of violent feelings and actions.

Here are some examples of these operations from my individual sessions in the psychiatric hosptial and group session in the Day training Centre for recidivists spoken about in Chapter 10.

---1a (The emotion both expressed musically and acknowledged). A young mother was panic-stricken because she shook all over, especially her hands, every time her first baby screamed. She had been very jealous of her younger sibling and this long-repressed feeling was now displaced on to her own child following the released flow of emotion generally in the form of maternal love. She had been to art therapy and showed me her painting of the monsters which she feared would attack her at night. We improvised on "Shaking" and "Monsters." She could feel the sadistic impulses which had been projected into these phantasy monsters and could understand the shaking partly as fear of them, and partly as a brake to stop them being carried out. This was a healthy linking up, and the beginning of her understanding of the jealous rage for which her own Inner Child had never found any acceptable outlet or acknowledgement. Also she was able to realise that she was not a Bad Mother, and these feelings had, in reality, nothing to do with her own mothering but could be worked through with understanding and without too much guilt as a resonance from the past.

---1b (Expressed musically but blocked intellectually). A young single woman was involved emotionally with the husband of another woman. She had lacked affectionate attention from her own father and had had to share the little there was with a number of siblings. We discussed this longing for an older man's affection and improvised to the title "Stealing the Father." Her xylophone music resembled a furtive running about, a true picture of the kind of lifestyle such relationships can bring with them. But she told me that she had no thoughts and feelings at all. She was anyway a patient who turned her emotion into psychosomatic symptoms; and the painful aspects and roots of this musical expression were not, at that point in her development, available to her.

This mode can also be linked to the fact that many offenders' crimes were committed in dissociation from their feelings of guilt. In psychotherapy the resistance vacuum is expressed as silence and it can be powerfully creative. But when music therapists can play the sound of the silence with their patients, we can reach the same results with less frustration and more immediate creativity arising directly from the matrix of the resistance vacuum.

---1c (Musical expression and strong aural impression). A young Caribbean offender played beautifully on the metallophone. We were doing a group improvisation on self-chosen colours. Others chose pink, green and yellow but he said simply: "I just like the sound of this instrument." This was his usual mode of operation. There was nothing wrong with it, it was perfectly straight-forward: playing is about sounds and listening to them. But the exercise was mixing imagination and music and it was interesting that this singly-focussed attention was his usual response. One day he chose to improvise as a cockatoo in the jungle. He made some exciting explorations into the musical possibilties of the piano but still could only talk about the quality of the sounds with nothing about his feelings or imagination sparked off by the music. Maybe he just chose to do this at this time as a right to privacy as against the request for personal sharing, or maybe he felt too threatened and needed to stick to the outer reality of the here-and-now. I don't know. In a short term group there is not always the time to explore one individual's motivation that deeply.

There may well be musicologists who say that their mode of operation is also always 1c. But then they are not in therapy where one is asked to explore one's feelings; and it is also possible that some of them may only be able to express emotion in music. With some hypersensitive children, music is frequently chosen as an alternative and more private way of expressing their emotion. They then keep severed the links between musical and verbal expression as a defence against intrusion into private, shame-donating and vulnerable aspects of themselves. For the same reason auditions, examinations or public performances can pose a very real unconscious threat to such young people's feeling of personal psychic security.

---2 (Musical expression of the resistance vacuum followed by association). A woman of forty, in one of the caring professions, felt that the motherly, caring part of herself could not meet her own needy Inner Child. There seemed to be a barrier between them. I asked her to try and express the feelings coming up by imagining herself being the "Barrier." We improvised on this theme and her music perfectly expressed the resistance vacuum. She could not find out exactly what this Barrier was, but was aware of tension and fear, and felt "faint and far away." The exercise seemed to elicit a depersonalisation defence.

Another woman, in her late thirties, came to her session with "nothing to say." Her mind was in a jumble, she said. We improvised on "Jumble" which revealed repetitive resistance vacuum music. However, following this her thoughts and feelings came flooding out.

She felt that people used her and that no one loved her for herself. By expressing the resistance in music the vacuum was made fecund.

---3 (The musical expression of the resistance energy). The grandmother of a young offender had died. She had brought him up and he wanted to attend her funeral. His father had forbidden him to do so and the son expressed his feelings about this by raging on the drum, with his body taut and face contorted, apparently in paroxysms of anger. However, when he finished playing, he said, with tears rolling down his cheeks: "I didn't feel anything." He had fallen into the resistance vacuum, where there was no link between emotion and thought. This might have seemed to be 1b but the beating was compulsive and his tears showed that he was in touch with his underlying grief.

Drawing from my own limited experience, it may be of interest to note which kind of patients had used each operation. I was working in the psychiatric hospital and the Day Training Centre for recidivists at the time.

1a was used by all types of patients excluding those who habitually used 1b. 1b was used by a great deal of offenders and sometimes conversion hysterics (people who expressed their feelings through their bodies). 1c was used only by Caribbean black offenders and one particularly defensive Probation Officer. This could, in fact, be a form of saying: "My feelings are none of your business and private to me" and as such can be understood and respected but I am sure that certain rather schizoid musicologists would also use this mode. 2 was used mainly by manic depressives and obsessional neurotics. 3 was used chiefly by conversion hysterics and hysterics.

These investigations are in no way conclusive in themselves, being so restricted, but they are presented as a further adumbration of Freud's personal discovery of music as a "port of entry." It is interesting to see how the powerful medium of music can put the psychic mechanism into states of excitation with different patterns according to the players' various cultures and stages of development.

Essay Eighteen

Times Of Stress And The
Opportunity For Maturation

Help given at times of particular stress can prevent breakdown and provide the direction for the effort that will lead to genuine maturation. The analytical music therapist has excellent opportunites of providing such help during the course of giving treatment to his patients. It is worth considering the kinds of stressors that a patient could have to contend with.

We can tell our outpatients not to multiply the obvious physical stressors such as thirst, hunger, infection, heat, cold and fatigue. Some of these are avoidable and some unavoidable, but the patient can be advised to not purposely multiply the stressors by, for example, staying out very late and getting chilled while being ill. Such advice would seem superfluous but it is surprising how many times patients can be found to be setting up an unnecessarily physically stressful situation for themselves when they already have a serious emotional disturbance. For example: a depressed woman was first thinking about going to bed at two in the morning at a time when she had to get up to go to work at seven. She carried a load of fatigue round all day which did not help her depression. Another patient cheerfully told me that she was eating nothing but three crispbreads a day. All her clothes were too small because she had proudly bought them when she had lost an unhealthy amount of weight prior to her illness. Such an impoverished diet could, of course, in time produce symptoms of apathy and confusion.

A special stress experienced by the person known to be a psychiatric patient is not being believed when she is telling the truth, especially about a physical condition. Two examples from real life are the outpatient whose reaction to prescribed drugs were causing fecal incontinence which had occurred several times in the street, to her acute distress, and made her fearful of going out anywhere. The general physician, who was probably stressed herself and not inclined to take the patient seriously, just said: "Oh, but it has never actually happened" and the patient left in despair. The second was an inpatient with influenza and a high temperature who was told to get up off her bed because psychiatric patients were not allowed to lie on their beds during the day. The idea that they could have two kinds of disorder did not seem to be allowable.

Although it is true that the psychiatric patient may live partly in the world of dreams, it is not a totally black or white situation. So although a colleague of mine was told by a psychiatrist to be wary of believing anything that patients told her, I have found that there is an equal danger in not believing anything that your patient tells you on the ground that she is mad and cannot be taken seriously. This makes it very difficult for the patient to relate usefully on the basis of facts that can be believed and usefully ameliorated, if not by the music therapist then perhaps by another member of the team.

As for psychic stressors of patients, the most important seems to be a lack of feedback in the form of meaningful and realistic validation. This could be missing from family, friends, workmates or other peers of some kind. Any kind of feedback is preferable to none. Thus a patient who takes an overdose as a cry for help can also be giving a cry for feedback from an undiscovered friendly world. This is especially so for the lonely bedsitter dweller who belongs to no groups and has no caring circle of friends. Such desperate behaviour can be a plea for the patient to be given confirmation that she really exists and is valuable to someone in a way that is meaningful to herself, even if a warm embrace would have been more welcome than a stomach pump given by a man in a white overall. The disturbed schizophrenic will sometimes burn herself with cigarette ends or scratch her arms just to feel the pain as a strange kind of affirmation of being.

Dr. D. W. Winnicott (in a lecture I attended) described how he treated a young boy whose stealing episodes could be traced back to the trauma of sitting on his depressed mother's lap as a toddler and receiving no feedback, let alone validation, from her sad and inward looking eyes. Dr. Winnicott said that the boy was able to reach back in time and find what it was that he had lost and had felt that he had to steal, in a symbolic way.

Everyone must be aware of the stress caused by the need for constant and often traumatic changes to which one must make readjustment without time for the assimilation of the emotional resonances that they cause. It can take many years, for example, for a man to work through the reactions to a war trauma. It was not until the Second World War that psychiatrists were employed to help soldiers with these problems as well as the selection, morale and organisation of the military forces.

It is not always realised, however, that for some people lack of stimulation can also be a stress. We are told that if an individual is immersed in a flotation tank with blood-heat water and with eyeshades and ear muffs on, the stress of this lack of stimulation from outside will bring on hallucinations for some, while others will actually pay to have the experience. Stressed out American University students who had experienced this situation experimentally refused a second trial even when they were to be paid handsomely for doing absolutely nothing.

To avoid the stress of understimulation, the therapist will help the patient to find her optimum stimulation level. One bright pregnant out-of-work violinist living abroad became depressed and apathetic when looking after her house, her violinist husband (who was working) and her three-year old twins. However, she rallied at once when she was asked to lead an orchestral ensemble nightly. Both the playing and the periods of rest in the darkness in the orchestral pit gave her the stimulation and the fallow periods to think creatively about what she could do in the house. She did the job quite adequately (I say this modestly as it was me) and even took the performance to royalty in her stride, and the apathy and depression vanished like smoke.

A woman of 55, ground down by her teaching job, which she did extremely well, became alive and dynamic when she added to this a four-year evening university degree course for which she had to do a great deal of extra work including studying for most of her week-ends. She obtained her degree with a 2.1 mark, which was an excellent result, and went on to battle her way into the stimulating world of the theatre where, when able to find work, the possibilities of enjoying positive feedback can be very encouraging indeed.

These women had found that their optimum levels of stimulation were higher than they had imagined; by taking on schedules that might break other women, they found fulfillment and added zest for life. This was only because the extra workload was meaningful enough to provide the energy to pull the residual routine jobs along with it. If either of them had been given an increased load of their original work they would probably have broken down. One could say that it is a stress not to have the opportunity to use one's talents in a personally meaningful way, whether professionally or as a hobby. Therefore it is important for the therapist to recognise whether a patient is understimulated, depressed or simply worn down by thinking in a circular fashion about an inner conflict.

In this connection, analytical music therapy can lead directly back to the springs of creativity both by allowing the continuous creation of musical form to clothe unverbalised emotions, and by freeing the energy bound up in previously unconscious images. Something is created out of nothing; from an urge, an impulse, an emotional pain or joy, sound patterns of pitch and rhythm emerge which link two people.   Communication about the previously incommunicable becomes possible even though it is at times chaotic, ungainly and tenuous. A statement is made, an affirmation of being; there is a reaching out in realisation of an inner state or experience. And when, through the ensuing words, the "I-am-here" realization is experienced, it may be possible for the patient to move on from this emotional point, to make a leap forward towards growth and maturation.

Certain external events can be trigger points which can cause dangerous reverberations through the patient's emotional life. These can be very personal and idiosyncratic events such as reactions to certain people or situations, or they can fall into a general pattern of bad reactions to such events as separation through estrangements, deaths, divorce, children leaving home and so on. Sometimes it is any significant change such as marriage, loss, success, failure, or transitional phases such as adolescence, the menopause, or change of home or job. For some, the most difficult trigger point is rejection by family, friends, employers, colleagues, audiences, clients, teenage children or even the withering of favourite plants or death of favourite pets which resonate unhappily for them. For many people it is anniversaries of sad or traumatic events which can bring on a sudden depression without the person realising why. In a lecture, other details of which escape me, we were even told that there was a dog who had an accident and for many years on that day slunk into a corner and shivered and whimpered without anyone finding out why for a long time.

One manic-depressive patient came into a very dangerous emotional state when, twenty-three years after her divorce, she met some people who knew of and spoke about the woman who had taken over her husband. They did not know anything about her previous connection to this woman. The patient had no one to whom she could speak about this, as at that time her therapist was away on holiday, and she became disturbed to the extent that she could not sleep, experienced racing thoughts and suffered quite unusually from indigestion. The loss of sleep and racing thoughts were quite serious symptoms for anyone suffering from her illness as they could presage a manic attack such as had put her into hospital in the past. When her therapist returned she had an analytical music therapy session and was astonished at the strength of her fury in decibels at this younger woman's overtaking of her husband, so many years after the event. She had the insight that it was because at that time she, herself, had had an unresolved oedipus complex and had identified with this young woman "thief" to the extent that she could not rebuff her and positively validate her own marriage. Instead she helplessly watched a projected part of herself play a destructive role in it; no doubt, at some level, obtaining some curious satisfaction from this.

This explosion of anger in sound began to create a source of neutralised energy which was subsequently used in building up her own life and work. She also realised why she had arranged her life so that there was no longer anyone that could be taken from her and at least began to wonder if this state could be modified.

Interviews for jobs are a recurring stress for the psychiatric patient, especially the first interview following their first hospitalisation. The therapist can be with them while they explore the various paths open to them. Should they reveal the illness and risk not being offered the job? If they do reveal their illness and get the job, they might be regarded as a curiosity, and with any slightly unguarded behaviour on their part be considered living proof of the dangers of abnormality. Or should they keep their psychiatric record to themselves? Then they risk having no one understanding to turn to if they should go through a period of particular stress on the job; they also risk the continual strain of dismissal if their secret should be disclosed, or if it is discovered that they had witheld this information.

Regrettably the professionals whose business it would be to help them find a job often do not realise that "unstressful" jobs like shelf-filling, packing and putting cotton wool swabs in plastic packets can be mind-blowingly stressful to an intelligent creative person. Because these jobs cannot anchor their imagination and creativity, they can free them up for just the kind of psychotic roaming that had brought them into hospital in the first place. What psychiatric patients need is a job which uses all their potentials but also offers them regular breaks for mild exercise and relaxation and possibly a few brief extra holidays, even if they must accept a pay cut to have this.

In analytical music therapy, improvising and talking about all this helps patients begin to come to terms with the fact of the psychiatric label. When they themselves begin to accept their condition and its label, it makes it easier for their employers to accept them should they decide to be frank about their illness. If they decide not to reveal it at least they are fully aware of the need for a source of support in their environment, someone or some group with whom they can be quite open and honest about their feelings and condition. Certainly some employers are very enlightened and understanding about psychiatric illness; some are even willing to take the ex-patient back with an initial period of part-time work and full pay; others will not take the ex-patient back. Certainly there is discrimination.

An ex-patient known well to me, who had had a serious nervous illness, somehow avoided answering questions about such illness on the application. The subject was also happily bypassed in the interview. She subsequently took on a job in a typing pool doing all the most difficult letters because she was regarded as one of the most competent and intelligent shorthand typists there. When she left to take further training, she asked the supervisor how they would have reacted if they were told that someone had a nervous illness. "Well, of course, we would not employ such a person, because it would not be fair to the other workers who would have to carry half her load," was the reply. The ex-patient lacked the courage to say that she had had three breakdowns and, far from being dependent on the other workers, had been taking on all the most taxing work. So that ex-patient learnt that keeping secrets can pay and the supervisor learnt nothing.

A patient in therapy can at least learn to see the matter from all sides before she makes her decision. She will face the fact that there is still a stigma attached to people who have had psychiatric illness and she may even find this discrimination in herself. One otherwise intelligent woman experiencing severe conversion symptoms, resisted seeking specialised help saying," I refuse to admit I'm a mental case." If she had been my patient we would have explored her attitude to such "cases." Most people have a "mad" part of themselves locked away, a part which can be mad in the American (angry) sense or which may contain repressed sadistic or omnipotent phantasies. This is the part which they project on to the psychiatric patients en masse in institutions; it forms the basis of their discrimination against such patients and against themselves if they become emotionally disturbed.

Of course, to a certain extent a sane measure of caution among employers is quite justified: you could not expect a person with manic-depression to be chosen to drive an express train, for example. A large proportion of psychiatric patients do have a some form of emotional immaturity in certain areas of life, and in these areas need extra support, which may or may not be available or desirable from their employers or colleagues. Being aware of this, many patients, as they get better, develop a reaction-formation to their dependency needs and refuse resolutely to depend on anybody. It is a dangerous brittle independence. Through their analytical music therapy work they make the discovery of the awareness of loneliness not as a crushing, paralysing force but as a spur towards seeking out new relationships. They look at me in astonishment and say, "I have discovered that I need people." But then there is the question of the optimum distance that they can accept from these new friends. Somehow, after therapy this is paradoxically both a little nearer and a little farther away than the distance they accepted before, which was often totally involved or not there at all.

A young woman in her early twenties, with anxiety neurosis and conversion symptoms, said at the beginning of her therapy that she would never get married nor have children. Such events were regarded as insuperably stressful. During her analytical music therapy treatment she fell in love with a married man older than herself, whose marriage was failing. Still she vowed that she would never get married. Her unconscious pull towards her father, whom she loathed consciously as a reaction-formation to her deeply unconscious childish wish for him as a husband, was worked through in music and in words. Her envy of her mother who had produced a very large family, three of whom were younger than the patient, made it unsafe for her to set herself up as a target for similar envy from others were she to become a wife and mother.

As she worked on the feelings and confronted the painful facts and difficulties of marrying a divorced man who had children by his first wife, her attitude to her own mother changed; she no longer thought of her as the repository of all wisdom and goodness, able to countermand the powers of darkness, but instead criticised her as a bad wife because the parental marriage was in a precarious state. At one level she agreed to marry her by-now-divorced man as a kind of substitute reparation to her father. She was replacing her mother at one remove and showing her the way these things ought to be done. But the actual marriage ceremony was felt to be an impassable barrier. Consciously she felt nothing but love for her fiance but unconsciously she felt otherwise as we can see in the following dream. She had, in reality, been invited to dine with her new employer but her fiance had forbidden her to go. That night she dreamt that her fiance was in pieces, except for a whole head, in a plastic bag which she carried over her shoulder. Later she talked about feeling "cut up" because he would not let her dine with her employer. The dream was a reversal, in it her fiance was the one that was cut up and his head was on her back.

At her next session she reported feeling claustrophobic in the car on the way to discuss the wedding with her mother but all right on the way back. We talked about her being the first and not the eldest of the many daughters to get married and rival the mother's status. She improvised on Wedding. She played, as usual, full pelt on the xylophone and said she felt happy and excited but sad about her nearest sister being absent. She ended up feeling more contented and serene.

After a holiday gap (she only came fortnightly anyway) the patient had been to buy her wedding dress with her mother and sisters and felt "floaty" as if walking up the aisle. We improvised "Up the Aisle." Initially, her music sounded timid and nervous then freely floating, but when I introduced the tune "Here Comes The Bride," she began to play fortissimo and to "kill" each note (stopping the vibration and resonance by hammering down without releasing the beater), while continuing playing was very fast and feeling panicky with a sensation of having a hole in the pit of her stomach. I then asked her to play as the "Church" with me playing as the "Wedding Couple," and she felt the Church as saying: "There go another couple, they'll have their ups and downs but I will be watching over them." She herself had insisted on a church wedding, although she was not a churchgoer; perhaps the church was seen as an alternative benign holding mother. She wanted to go with her sister and say a prayer before the wedding in church. On one level I will accept that a prayer is a prayer is a prayer but there could have been an element of magical protection against envy in this one. The wedding went off smoothly except for one small, manageable palpitation in the vestry. But the patient was disappointed that not enough fuss was made of her, not enough cuddling and admiration.

In facing up to this stressful time the patient struggled and grew to a point of greater maturity, facing up to her jealousy, which I have not discussed here, originally of her younger siblings, now of her husband's children and mother, of her fear of envy and of the guilt caused by the unconscious incestuous feelings about wanting to steal a father from his wife and family. These underlying feelings were uncovered for the patient but the decision to go through with this wedding was nevertheless there. It was especially important that the patient made great strides forward during this difficult and demanding transition, as weddings are traditionally befogged by idealisation and the denial of any kind of negative feeling. Such immature standpoints are apt to recoil causing grief and bewilderment.

A forty year old manic-depressive woman felt extremely insecure in situations where she did not know what was going to happen. After several years of therapy two such situations arose at once. She was about to join a very active religious organisation with a commitment to a comprehensive set of rules, and at her new job the man who had been a good boss suddenly disappeared without her understanding why. She was surrounded by unknowns. We played

some music about "Uncertainty." She built up her part using first one
then two, three, four and five beaters. The music started with a bleak
emptiness that was unusual for her. Gradually it became richer and
more confident.

In spite of the fact that I felt that the disappearing boss might
hold reverberations from the time when her soldier father left home,
she said that she felt that both situations held out opportunities for her
and that she would be able to manage to use them. Formerly she had
said, "How can I trust God when I can't trust people?" Now she could
manage to trust in her own growing to meet the needs of these
situations and this showed real maturation.

Usually reactions to a particular psychic stressor develop in a
predictable cycle. At first the patient is overwhelmed by her reaction
to a situation and does not realise that this will be a recurring event.
Next this is pointed out to her and she is able to see it coming and say,
"Here I go again," without, however, being able to do anything about
it. The point of maturation comes when she sees the situation as a
danger and manages to survive by using some internal or external
means to help herself. In fact, this is usually finding a means to
comfort and steady the wounded "Inner Child" in herself. The patient
last quoted found some trust in her inner resources to overcome the
panic and anxiety that usually overwhelmed her in similar situations.

At any time, but particularly in times of stress, it is important
for the analytical music therapist not to fall into the trap of avoiding
the full amount of anxiety, anger or other negative feeling that the
patient may entertain, and suggest improvisation titles with magical
solutions. This is not to say that these feelings need to be forced out
of the patient when she is in a state of near-shock and needs first to
have help in getting her body's rhythm systems back to normal
functioning. But these feelings need not, therefore, be pushed under
the carpet in the hope that they will disappear or in the pretence that
they were never there. The therapist must be sensitive to their need
for an outlet when the time is ripe and the patient feels strong enough
to transmute them into something constructive and helpful in the
attainment of her positive life aims.

For an example, an Intertherapy student in the patient role,
wept at the sight of the Pope ministering to the masses in Ireland on

television. The therapist student-partner then suggested that he imagine meeting such a father (the patient's own father had been away a lot and had also been very occupied with his profession). Thus they bypassed all the feelings of sadness and deprivation. It was with these feelings that the patient needed helpful support and empathic understanding and had he left the therapy without getting this might well feel doubly alone and oppressed in his Inner Child subpersonality.

When these students switched roles another "magical" solution was prescribed. The student patient said that she felt overwhelmed by people and felt unable to "carve out" her own space. The therapist student suggested that they improvise on carving out her space which they did with dismal results. The patient felt that this was an impossible task for her. Whereas if they had improvised on the feelings about being overwhelmed and smothered, it is likely that her anger would have successfully completed the carving-out process. She might also have had an insight into the original root of the feeling of having this space disallowed, thus making it seem easier to overcome at an adult level.

One of the calculated stresses of the therapy situation is the lack of gratification. But it is just this stress that drives the patient out into life to arrange for gratifications there in the form of true two-way friendships, work that is rewarded, creativity which is longer-lasting, satisfying sexual relationships and the sharing of food, drink and talk.

However, if there is not given some subtle hint to the patient that she is lovable, that her creativity is valuable and her work is rewardable, her personality may be withered in the bud as it were, and she will in identification cease to nourish herself with any hope that things could ever be different and stop trying. Nevertheless total gratification of this kind within the session is seduction from life and makes life the impossible stress which must be defended against rigorously until the next gratifying session comes along. Therefore it is so necessary to have some real knowledge of the patient's outer life in its various aspects as well as what goes on in the session.

Although one is recommended not to see patients outside the session, I have always found it enormously useful to see the patient in other situations and with other people. This was easily done in the hospital where I worked for twenty years, as the patient might also be in the choir, or taking the role of hostess in the Music Club, and where one also had feedback from the multidisciplinary team. In my experience what most patients had hidden from the therapist was usually their strengths but this is not always the case. Some will make gigantic and sometimes tragically successful efforts to hide a weakness from their therapist.

The therapist must be able to face the stress of realising his non-omnipotence (I will not say impotence). He cannot give the patient the rewards and good experiences that she must look for in life but he can offer her companionship on some of the darker roads and help her to forge the weapons to fight the shadowy creatures that she may meet there. He can also be her companion in success when she may have to face withering and often baffling envy for the first time.

Times of stress, viewed as opportunities for maturation, can produce in both therapist and patient the incentive to struggle and grow.

Essay Nineteen

Analytical Music Therapy And The "Detour Through Phantasy"

This essay is based on a talk originally given at the 1979 Conference of the British Society for Projective Psychology and Personality Study. Its title contains a phrase, "The Detour Through Phantasy," which captured me as I was reading Heinz Hartmann's Ego Psychology and the Problem of Adaptation (1958). Here is the complete quotation: "Taking our point of departure from pathology, from the psychology of neuroses and psychoses, we come to overestimate the positive developmental significance of the shortest pathways to reality, and it is only when we set out from the problem of reality adaptation that we recognise the positive value of the detour through phantasy."

A phrase like that tends to capture us when we have a body of experience which cries out to be neatly clothed in its verbal skin. The body of experience was, in this case, some work in my private analytical music therapy practice which constituted a detour---in fact several detours---through phantasy. We, the patients and I, took these detours without any conscious knowledge that this might be the best way as regards reality-adaptation; we took them because they seemed to be the only routes open to us at the time. In the case that follows it was necessary for me to enter the patient's phantasy world because she was unable, at that time, to enter the challenging world of more generally accepted reality.

I wondered what it would be like to make this detour purposively, and decided to call on a colleague to make an improvisation with me to the title of this chapter. As the therapist, she sat at the hospital Steinway grand piano and I sat, as the patients do, behind a battery of instruments comprising an alto chromatic xylophone, a 16" tom-tom, a gong and a cymbal. There were other smaller instruments nearby: a melodica, double naqqaras, a chordal dulcimer - that sort of thing. (At home I also have a home-made bell-tree with bells from all over the world).

We started playing, and immediately I found myself in a leafy jungle running for my life with a horde of angry psychologists after me. I was thudding along on the xylophone and annihilating the strident sounds of my colleague's pianistic cacaphony with the drum and cymbal. A slightly paranoid impression of my talk to the Projective Psychologists and a timely warning to me not to get too defensive at question time. My colleague felt that the title gave her carte blanche to pull out all the stops of musical creativity and fantasy. Having made this experiment with myself as patient, I felt confident to try it out on my patient.

Curtis (as I will call him) was referred to me by a consultant psychotherapist with the words: "It is either music therapy or nothing!" Curtis was a tall, pleasant but anxious-faced thirty-two year-old man of medium build. He had recently been hospitalised with schizophrenia and was still falling into catatonic states and finding speech difficult. He lived then with his parents, being recently divorced but without children. His father, with whom he had a poor relationship, was a professional man and Curtis had been studying for the same profession until he cut loose, left this country, married a dancer from the Continent, taught English and studied singing, only to be told that he had insufficent talent to become a professional musician.

At the time therapy commenced, he was working behind the scenes with people in a commercial concern, a job that his mother had helped him to obtain. (How he coped I could not imagine. Certainly there had been a very poor report on his work just before we started therapy). He had a sister some years older who was married and had five children, and Curtis had a good relationship with that family. He was quite cut off from any of his former friends and led a restricted life working, chatting sparsely to his parents, watching television, and retiring to bed early. Here he listened to the radio (what else he did he did not say); certainly he was unable to read at that time.

Curtis came for treatment in early spring. I had comprehensive notes on his case from his consultant psychiatrist and the referring consultant psychotherapist, but I always like to have the patient's own version of his story to see how it has been edited for me and how it felt from the inside. I wrote in my notes that he seemed dim and faint; his hold on reality seemed as fragile as a soap bubble. He could not initiate speech but answered monosyllabically when asked a question, seemingly in some distress. After a brief history-taking we moved quickly on to the instruments.

We played together for ten timed minutes. He played quietly but with interest, mostly on the xylophone. Afterwards I explained that we were going to record the next improvisation and the microphone would not pick up such quiet playing. We then improvised on his imagined "Mountain Climb." He made a quiet start then came rain and thunder on the drums, the sun coming out with cymbal and glissandi on the xylophone, climbing up and crossing the stream, and resting under a tree. I thought that this symbolised this stage of his life when he was protected by his family. Then he went on and climbed to the top but imagined no view. When he told me about his visualisation he spoke clearly, his face flushed and his eyes much brighter. There was a countertransference of sadness.

The "Mountain Climb" theme was an exercise used by Dr. R. Assagioli (1965) to discover a patient's life aspiration. I decided not to discuss the possible meaning of Curtis' phantasy in reality terms. I felt that he was too frail to make such connections for the moment, just as in our talk, I had to be the model for a fluently communicating person rather than subjecting him to the stress of long, tense silences when his words would not form themselves. Fifteen months later, I was sometimes empty and silent to receive his verbal flow, and sometimes responding and amplifying, too, like a good musical instrument.

For the first eleven sessions (once-weekly for an hour), we vacillated between fantasy and reality in our titles. There were, in fact, five phantasy titles and six reality titles. The fantasy titles were: "Mountain Climb" (he chose to do this three times, each time differently), "The Castle of the Self," and "The Dream at Work." These titles were fruitful in that they seemed to cause a release of energy and expression in music and more especially in words. But, possibly because I thought we ought to be exploring the shortest pathways to reality, they were interspersed with titles of: "The Artist versus the Professional," "Mother," "Holiday," "Father," "Conversations at Work," and "Dr. F" (his consultant psychiatrist). These last, though fruitful, seemed to stop the flow of free verbal expression and to block him and give him a sad, perpelexed look as if he had been deprived suddenly and inexplicably of something that he loved.

If phantasy was what released him and set him free to communicate, then I decided that we would resolutely turn our explorations that way and see where it led. I was interested to provide a title that might lead to the exploration of his aggressive and sexual drives.

In his twelfth session he told me that he was now able to deny accusations at work. His speech was more fluent with fewer of the former helpless gestures which had pleaded to be magically understood like the preverbal baby with the good-enough mother who preserves just a little of his illusion of omnipotence.

We took the title "Finding the Dagger in the House." He imagined going up the front stairs, standing waiting in front of the door, then going downstairs into a room looking out on to trees, seeing a jewel-encrusted dagger and a bowl of fruit. He thought of eating the fruit but left both fruit and dagger and came away. I said that living at home was rather like eating the fruit and leaving the dagger. His music started in a rapid quaver 4/4 beat which sounded first urgent and then questing as he changed to crotchet and quaver beats and lead finally into a stale repetitive pattern. This seemed to point to his domestic situation where the home comforts (breast/fruit) with mother demanded the sacrifice of the use of the dagger/penis of tough thinking. I hoped for something more archaic, and in the next session, after we had played our ten minutes untitled duet and an improvisation in the Aeolian mode, we improvised with the title "Finding the Sword in the Forest." His music started out in a brisk 6/8, it was lively and rhythmically varied with drumming, careful use of cymbal and free xylophone glissandi. He imagined going up a hill to the forest, hearing birds singing, seeing flowers blooming, coming to a river where the sword lay dirty and out of its scabbard. He cleaned it and buckled it on to himself and went on his way. The countertransference was of madness which I played while he continued as his determined and purposeful self.

Next session our title was "After Getting the Sword." He imagined that he went uphill to a deep forest with rocks sticking out of the ground and found a white, turreted castle where a White Lady lived with her maidens. They gave him a meal and in some mysterious way he pledged his services to her (this bit was played very quietly, almost reverently). He also glanced at me when he said this as if I were the lady in question. The music was full of purpose and most moving with an almost sacramental intimacy in places.

He came an hour early for the next session. His ten minute improvisation took on an eager speed; he improvised a song about a flower that grew and grew while I drummed on the tambour. Next we took the title "After the White Castle." He imagined that he got up, had breakfast and the White Lady told him to fetch the stag from a mountain forest. He found the way up the mountain, and in a clearing saw the herd with playful fauns. He lassoed the stag and on the way home it swam the river ahead of him. The music was at first a nonchalant, pleasant 6/8 but became more urgent in the middle of the piece and had more emotional range. He looked sharper and more in focus when we finished. All these vivid inner experiences contrasted sharply with his apathetic everyday appearance and experience.

In the next session we did our ten minute improvisation in an ABA form as I thought he needed some conscious creativity to balance the phantasies. Our title was "After the Stag." The White Lady told him to go to a tower and fetch the book inside. He had to cross a river and the tower was guarded by a dragon which he discouraged with a wooden pole. He brought the book back without looking in it. The music started with gentle downward glissandi and had dynamism and character. He told his story with fluency and conviction.

The dragon seemed to represent the negative aspect of the White Lady, an archetypal smothering, all-devouring and womb-imprisoning mother. He could well have connected this with his infantile fears regarding his own mother as he looked so shocked and pained when I asked if he had killed it. I remarked on the suppression of his curiosity regarding the book and wondered privately if his epistomophilic instinct was in the service of his mother rather than himself.

During this time Curtis attended his hospital one evening a week for a Social Skills group; he always spoke about this and we incorporated the teaching into our work where it seemed relevant. I thought that this strong outpouring of unconscious material should be subjected to as much conscious scrutiny as possible (thinking of Jung's recommendation to this affect); and in the absence of a qualified art therapist I asked him to make some coloured pictures of the story so far, the accent being more on the effort to bring these images into the world of everday than on the end product.

In the seventeenth session he arrived with the first three of the chalk drawings of the tale; they were primitive but quite strong. We played "After the Book." He imagined that he set out from the castle to find the bugle that was the horn of an animal. There was a storm in the night. He came to an encampment and played draughts with a man and won the horn. He blew it and brought it back. His speech was enthusiastic and fluent. He had been to concerts and theatres in his holiday and looked well.

At the next session we finished this personal myth. It seemed to come to a natural end. We improvised "After the Bugle." The White Lady read in the book that he was to take the stag to another herd where it must fight the existing leader and take over. And this was done. The music was quite stormy and emotional and there was some interesting musical dialogue, which seemed to indicate that I had suddenly become a separate person for him to play with and not just a part of his larger self. There was a countertransference of anger which I expressed freely, and he drummed acceptance of it. It is interesting how patients accept countertransference expression if the moment for the transmission of the emotion from the unconscious is right. Either they freeze at the sound of a melody which expressed their deepest, most secret self and play pianissimo while it lasts, or they play along with more turbulent music if it seems somehow right to them. In the first case they will usually remark on the tune afterwards. One patient said: "That music was me." But such happenings are rare and very beautiful. The second kind of acceptance is more common.

But to return to Curtis and his detour through phantasy. This personal myth enabled him to begin to come to terms with his sexual and aggressive drives which were never expressed crudely but always wrapped in the symbolism of the sword, the tower, the stag with erect horns and the bugle made from an animal's horn. Overcoming his father, in the Oedipal sense, was symbolised by the winning of the game of draughts, the vanquishing of the stage leader and taking the phallic sword from the genital river in the archaic forest mother's depths. The mother/wife was split into the White Lady - quite a demanding woman in her way - and the dragon guarding his access to the book of knowledge in the tower; which he overcame with the aid of a long pole. The pledging of his service to the White Lady had the quality of a sacrament, there was an almost tangible feeling of deep mystery while he played this passage. I wondered if the music made the myth possible or did the myth produce the music, or were they mutally creative? I am inclined to believe the last.

Being firmly lodged in reality and relationship through our music, Curtis could safely have access to and share his phantasy. This phantasy indeed resembled a psychic nature reserve, as Freud described in his Complete Works (Volume 16): "The mental realm of phantasy is just such a reservation withdrawn from the reality principle" (p. 372).

As the therapist I played the part of a super-ego milder than his own, which allowed him to contact this inner world. I made almost no interpretations because I felt that his ego was as yet too fragile to tolerate them. Transference interpretations, in particular, I believed would have jarred him too brutally out of his world of phantasy and perhaps made it difficult for him to distinguish the boundaries between his inner and outer worlds. Nevertheless there was a link, through music therapy, between his phantasy nature reserve and the world of outer reality. To quote Freud again: "There is a path that leads back from phantasy to reality - the path, that is, of art."

At that time a positive idealised mother transference was casting the White Lady projection on to me, but I was ready and willing to be cast in the role of the obfuscating dragon at any time. Curtis was unable, at the start of this therapy, to work out a man-to-man relationship with his father. He had totally abandoned all competition with him through his original profession but through phantasy he felt that he was able to master the tasks of manhood and that gave him more confidence in reality in connection with his work and relationships. His music had been changing too; he was bolder rhythmically, more creative with melody and more adventurous in expressing a wider range of emotion. But it still had mainly a synthetic or synthesizing function, keeping his psyche together while he experienced this tenuous connection between inner and outer worlds.

Three months after the myth ended, Curtis moved out of his parents' home and into a mixed hostel and was cooking, shopping, washing and ironing for himself and loving it. For his aggressive impulse towards his parents, expressed in the vanquishing of the stag and dragon, he made reparation by taking on sparetime voluntary work taking an old lady out in her wheelchair. He regained his gentle sense of humour; he was able to read once more and filled the rest of his leisure with the pursuit of the pleasant, in the form of visits to films, plays, concerts and art galleries and dining out with one or two friends. Altogether I felt that his detour through phantasy had returned quite generously to reality.

The Inner Child

Whatever chronological age your analytical music therapy patient is, you are always partly working with the child she once was. For the past is not over and done with, but lives on in the present person, affecting every mood and every decision and every relationship. One can think of the personality as being like the trunk of a tree, which when sawn down, reveals the meagre growth of poor years and the rich growth of the good years, and all these together constitute the sum total of the tree's being at any given time.

According to Dr. Culver Barker (1972), there are two kinds of hurt which can freeze part of the personality at the child level. One is a trauma such as the death of a parent, a hospitalisation or a sexual seduction. Of course what constitutes a trauma for one child may not affect another at all or may even have a beneficial effect. He cites the case of a little boy who went into hospital and was called "a little hero" by the surgeon and came out bursting with confidence and vitality. Traumas are believed by some to be caused by reality providing a confirmation of a terrifying phantasy. They are experiences which the individual cannot assimilate and therefore are mastered by the use of energy-depleting defences.

Another kind of damage is caused by the prevailing emotional climate in which a child grows up. It may be an atmosphere of coldness with a schizoid mother, or a critical, complaining atmosphere which kills all affection, a long battle over toilet-training or a stifling overprotection which withers all spontaneity, curiosity and adventure. Whatever it is, the child who suffered it, lives on in the adult.

For example, I treated a patient who hated birthdays, not because the advancing years were taking their toll of her looks, as she was still in her early twenties, but because a birthday held a forgotten, bitter memory.

In her musical improvisation we explored her first, second, third amd fourth birthdays with nothing but happy memories of friends and cakes and presents and candles. When we came to the fifth birthday things were very different. She was put in touch with feelings about a sad day when her nursemaid was suddenly (or so it seemed to

her) given the sack by her father. The patient had been very attached
to her and remembered with pleasure that the nursemaid had shown her
all her dresses. The memory was of a moment of hurt and bewilderment when the nursemaid was no longer there at her birthday tea.
Although she had forgotten this until our improvisation, it had caused
a shadow and the expectation of sadness and disappointment to fall on
subsequent birthdays.

Another patient, when eight years old, reacted badly to being
forbidden entrance to her home and mother by her grandmother during
her mother's confinement. The patient had been sent to stay with
neighbours. The situation had been so traumatic for her that she
repeatedly stage-managed similar situations in the present when she
expressed a fury that was out of all proportion to the present situation.
During her stay at the psychiatric hospital where I worked she became
furious and violent when she was shut out of the Sister's office during
the psychiatrist's visit. Much later, I said that she could not always be
sure of contacting me during the weekend if she felt suddenly
depressed but that she could always contact the Samaritans. She was
very angry about this, stirring up a whole army of well-meaning
helpers in between our sessions who all gave her different kinds of
good advice, ending with her being sent off on holiday to the coast and
missing her next session with me. In fact for a depressed patient on
her own, taking a holiday is often the worst thing she could be advised
to do as the guilt this produces can even lead to suicidal attempts,
whereas working can use up the energy of residual underlying anger.

That patient could not remember the shock that she had felt at
being shut out and then finding when she was allowed home that she
had apparently been replaced by an adored howling red baby---a boy
at that. So she would continually act out the situation in the present to
try and relieve the frozen emotion. Each time she did this the root
cause had to be pointed out to her. The repetitions became less
frequent as we worked, but still would occur at awkward and unexpected moments and have to be interpreted once again. Their irrational
quality of childish rage and stubbornness made them extremely hard to
deal with even for the therapist and patient. For others unwittingly
involved they had the flavour of frightening and violent madness. But
it helped me to realise that though I seemed to be working with an

adult, I was actually in touch with the unhealable wound of an angry, baffled and painfully jealous child of eight who felt suddenly and miserably unloved and rejected. It is possible that such violent emotion could be better helped for a period by a more body-based holistic therapist who could allow for their release with ensuing physical relaxation through whole-body kicking and raging and also some physical holding to call up the early safe and pleasurable feelings of being the baby, through the kinaesthetic rather than the more rarified musical experience.

The actual time when such damage takes place Dr. Barker called "the point of critical hurt." Sometimes this point takes place very early, at a time when the child is not yet able to speak or even think in words. Yet the music improvised with the patient can bring back vivid memories mostly of touch, sights, and strong feelings of being loved or not loved.

One patient was getting attacks of dissociated violence when she would smash cups and windows and want to set fire to the curtains and hurl herself in front of trains or cars. She had a good working alliance with me and we discussed the need for her adult part to contain these angry child feelings even though this might be experienced as quite painful and difficult. We improvised some music about "Holding." She played long quiet notes on the melodica, and had the inner experience of feeling that a soft blanket was being drawn round her in a loving way. I felt that she was reaching right back to a time when she had really felt lovingly held and contained by her mother, and I felt motherly towards her. Her own mother was often depressed and had probably left her feeling quite desperate at times, as she described in another session "..dissolving and evaporating like drops of water in the sun." The week after the blanket experience she did feel more able to contain her aggressive impulses, though she was very frightened of them. She was also able to get in touch with and express physically a terrible knot of pain inside herself, wailing like a small child in an abandonment of misery. In her case the source of this hurt was something that neither of us could find words for, but through the music I shared with her a deep sadness.

Because these points of critical hurt live on in patients in the present, they colour certain aspects of their lives, often making them unpredictable and difficult to live with unless their companions have extraordinary patience, tolerance and understanding.   However, sometimes through therapy they can gradually absorb and assimilate the formerly unassimilable experience usually with much fear and emotional pain. During this period of the work, the patient will need the greatest support by the therapist and also a lot of support from the environment. That means that the carers will have to be cared for too. Failing this she may briefly have to go into hospital which is sometimes a helpful experience in spite of the stigma and lack of the basic needs for fresh food, clean air and daily exercise. The terror of the trauma seems to be greater when the damage was done to the patient when she was preverbal.   The fear then is of something nameless, formless, and infinitely terrible because it cannot be contained by thoughts.

These resonations of early terrors are very contagious and often affect those near to the patient with an intense fear of her as a person. Even therapists can sometimes feel their own unworked-through infantile fears activated by patients in this state, and it is thus easy for scape-goating to occur in the immediate environment.

The patient, if enabled to do so, is often helped by experiencing and expressing physically the emotion that was frozen at the point of critical hurt. But this is only helpful if it can then be integrated at adult level. However, some people in caring professions have adapted to the inner child situation in a different way. Early on they have found that it was too painful to contain their own inner child so they have taken up a profession through which they could project this part of themselves into a client and look after it there. In this way they are likely to become very involved with their clients and find themselves working seven days a week and at all hours to cope with the demands made upon them. They really feel that they cannot say no to anyone, or refuse to aid desperately projected parts of themselves. In this way many members of caring professions are burnt out, and eventually have to have some help for themselves in coming to grips with their own Inner Child. Professionals in the caring professions who have this built into their training have a better chance of survival. Even if the early traumatic situation is not totally worked through at that time, the worker knows that acceptable help is possible, and if she starts to feel overwhelmed by a situation is not afraid of reaching out for more professional help.

A schoolteacher who came to me for analytical music therapy, said that before she started therapy she was especially interested in the sad misfits in her class and spent a great deal of time with them. After about two years of treatment she did not feel that she wanted to get unnecessarily attached to them in any way, she had enough to deal with in coping with her own Inner Child feelings. But later on she became interested in one very angry child and this was in the months preceding the emergence of a very aggressive, partly dissociated part of herself. Once more she felt that she could not deal with anyone else who was angry, and when she was hospitalised she left the ward for some days because she felt that she was getting too involved with a violent, manic patient. Each time she began to work with the bruised feelings of her own Inner Child, she withdrew that projection from the children she worked with and felt that she no longer had the resources to deal with them while she was working with her own feelings.

Working through these Inner Child feelings with the above-mentioned patient, one day she told me that she had been having a "worried" feeling which became more and more intense until she began to float off in a strange dreamy state which was most unpleasant and did not seem to resolve anything. She seemed to be using a psychotic mechanism for defence against experiencing the full impact of this inner anxiety. We decided to explore this in music. I felt quite secure in doing this as at this moment she was staying in hospital and would not have the hour-long journey home on her own in what might possibly be an unsteady state of mind---or rather emotion. We called the improvisation "The Worried Feeling." She began with a long and very intense crescendo on the 16" tom-tom. I felt the tremendous power in her music come to a kind of crossroads inside me. On one side was the holding which I was doing with massive major chords, on the other side was this tremendous feeling of anxiety. At last her music reached a climax and she played on the xylophone with a confident sound. When we had finished, the patient said she had felt the worried feeling growing greater and greater but at the same time she felt completely held by my music, and suddenly she felt like a tiny child held and wrapped safely round in a shawl. Then she felt she had grown out of that and wanted to grow up and at the end she felt we were equals. Following this she faced a long weekend alone at home with considerable confidence. The tricky part for the therapist is to be able, like lightning, and at the exactly right moment, to allow the patient to be at what age she needs to be and not hold her back in a strangling cocoon.

It seemed that this patient used this psychotic mechanism of dreamy, unreal states of mind to defend herself from the unassimilated peaks of suffering, some of which she was experiencing belatedly and with terror and bewilderment in the present. Before this inner child subpersonality began to emerge she used to sit crouched forward, hiding behind her long, brown hair, often crying and letting her nose drip like the uncared-for child. Since the emergence of this sub-personality she sat with her face bared and took care of the drips on her nose with the proffered tissues. The caring and cared-for parts were beginning to come together and she was gradually able to be a caring mother to the wounded child inside herself.

A student in training, undergoing Intertherapy, came to her session talking a lot and rather denigratingly about her father. At the same time she brought a dream which she had had when she was three, and which she remembered because she had always felt it was very important to her. First she told how, when she had stood by a river or the sea, her father would always say: "If you fall in I won't be able to pull you out." In the dream she stood with her parents by a river of thick brown mud in a completely brown landscape where even the sky was brown. She put a foot in the mud and was sucked in, pulling one parent in who then pulled the other one in.

With her student partner she improvised her feelings about the dream. Her head was thrown back with her eyes closed and tears streaming down her cheeks as she beat the gong and cymbal as if she would destroy the whole world. Her partner did a masterful job of holding her with the piano music. She never let go for a minute. When the client student had finished, she said she had been walking alone in a desert of mud, feeling that she was going on alone even into eternity. She had been followed by sounds that came and went and were very threatening to her, but not dangerous. Later she said that she wanted to be alone; it was better that way. She mentioned in passing that she had shared her parent's bedroom until she was three.

We saw the brown landscape as her infantile omnipotent destructive feelings accompanying defecation; and her furious jealousy at hearing the parents' intercourse in their big bed. Because of this overwhelming jealousy, she felt that she must always be alone as if she had a partner she could risk facing from someone else the furious destructive jealousy that she herself had aimed at her parents. And after the disappointment of realising that, in spite of the exciting game in the parents' bed which she and her younger sister had had, her father belonged only to her mother sexually. She defended herself against this disappointment by a sour grapes attitude, calling father a weak and therefore undesirable man.

This student fell right back into her inner child experience; this subpersonality took over wholly as she cried and raged like an infant. However, she managed to resurrect her adult self in order to be the therapist to her partner, though she was crying again on her journey home.

Usually the presence of the inner child makes itself known through the material the patient presents. But when this is not the case and the therapist suspects the presence of damaged child subpersonality, he can use various techniques to bring out some of its feelings. One of these is to let the patient and himself alternate in playing Child and Adult. In this way the patient may be put in touch with her possible projection into an outside child or animal. She may be able to discover what child or animal when she herself takes the Child role.

Another technique involves asking the patient to imagine standing in a house at the top of some dark steps leading to a cellar and calling "Is there anyone there that needs me?" Here the cellar represents the unconscious. Sometimes the patient's unconscious will produce an imaginary child figure which will converse with her. Sometimes she may suddenly feel that she is that child figure herself, in other words she will regain the consciousness of that child subpersonality. Not every technique brings results with every patient. Symbolic imagery produces striking effects with some patients but others do not relate this way to their unconscious at all.

Most of the techniques in analytical music therapy were developed in response to a particular patient's needs and tried out first in my own Intertherapy trio with Marjorie Wardle and Peter Wright, my colleagues at that time.   There is nothing to stop any working music therapist developing their own techniques to suit their own personality, temperament and patients.

Music can often help to make these deep emotional experiences available to the conscious mind. Temporarily, of course, the last state can seem worse than the first because the net result is suffering. But conscious suffering does not produce the symptoms and psychotic states of mind caused by suppression of the unexpressed suffering frozen into the individual's child subpersonality and unknown to its owner.   The freeing expression of the music, together with the physical tears and raging, are part of the very exhausting but healing process. With the physical expression of this emotion together with the understanding of its origins and meaning comes a relaxation which the client can find wonderfully freeing as defences against sobbing and raging are expressed somatically as permanent energy-depleting tensions or "muscle armours" in the body.

For the analytical music therapist, the knowledge and healing of his Inner Child through the unfreezing of its traumatised emotion, are an essential part of his inner preparation for work. In this way he will make sure of treating his patients as separate individuals without causing them to express the emotions of his unconscious and projected damaged inner child instead. However, the healing process seldom ends dramatically with the expression of emotion; for client or patient it must also go on to the practice of the taking over of the mothering of her own wounded Inner Child, so that she does not burden her near and dear ones with this tedious role.

Essay Twenty-One

Affirmations And Celebrations

Most of the time in analytical music therapy, the therapist and patient are exploring together, patiently pushing back the barriers of the unknown. It is hard work. It can be very magnetising. I think that is the right word rather than exciting---but often it is also painful for the patient and uncomfortable for the therapist. On the other hand, during this exploration they come to psychic places which can be likened to oases in the desert. Once here they do not push on any more for the moment, but pause and consolidate their gains. This is done through improvising affirmations or celebrations. Celebration is described in Chambers 20th-Century dictionary as "to distinguish by solemn ceremonies" and "to publish the praise of." Where one would use wine and a toast, and possibly a libation, the therapeutic couple use music. The ceremony is indeed sometimes solemn but it can also be hilarious; and always it registers with the patient as: "This was worthy of attention, we celebrated!"

All over the world there are sayings which warn against hubristic celebration such as the English "Don't count your chickens before they are hatched" or the French "Do not keep your holidays until they arrive." If a forthcoming cause for celebration is announced, the phrases "Touch wood" or "D.V." are often added to ward off Hubris, the ancient Greek sin of presumption. In the past one libated to the gods not only to honour them but also to ward off their envy. These envious gods and spirits were in reality the parent figures who were experienced as envious because the impotent infant projected his own tremendous envy into them and then introjected them as equally envious and potentially destructive inner objects.

In Envy and Gratitude, Melanie Klein (1975) wrote: "The super-ego figure on which strong envy has been projected becomes particularly persecutory and interferes with thought processes and with every productive activity, ultimately with creativeness."

Therefore candidates for celebrations must be selected a bit carefully. If they, themselves, are unconsciously strongly envious, they may be too fearful of being made enviable to allow any celebration to take place. In fact one or two of my patients have anxiously refused a celebratory improvisation, clearly on this ground, though they were not aware of it. So it is necessary for the celebrant to be able to withstand a certain amount of envy.

If, on the other hand, the patient is a person whose defence against envy is to become as enviable as possible, then the celebration may be adding fuel to the feelings of persecutory anxiety which such actions arouse.

With the depressive type of patients whose defence against rivalry is to devalue themselves, the celebration can provide the courage to endeavour to live up to their full potential with the sense of the therapist as an ally. Often I have not been aware of a patient's fear of envy until I have seen their reaction to a mooted celebration.

A teacher in his late twenties had suffered a manic-depressive episode. After a year back at work he had accepted a promotion but denied its importance as a tribute to his work, partly, I felt, as a defence against a manic explosion of triumph. His "Celebration of Promotion" was quite quiet, mezzopiano, figures jumping up in pitch as usual and the petering out with a kind of warning cymbal growl. I told him that people who had been manic often at first could not trust themselves to celebrate. He said that when he got out of school on the day when he had been told of his promotion, he had felt like doing something completely wild; but he had been told to keep it to himself and as there was no one there anyway who would understand just how he felt, he did nothing. Several weeks later he did let slip that he had quite an ambitious plan for studies that should lead to further and more satisfying causes for celebration.

Patients present one with their bitter memories of the lack of any celebration at key moments in their young lives. The parents who provided these bleak moments were often more worried about their own value. Though they may have seemed unimaginative and unempathetic they may not have been as envious as their offspring felt them to be. A patient who had started learning the violin at fourteen, won a scholarship at a leading music college at eighteen. The family was quite well off and the girl fully realised that scholarship money was for the deserving poor, but nevertheless her mother's reception of it: a non-congratulatory "We'll have to give the money back," which was not ameliorated in any way by her father, was felt by her daughter as an envious robbery of her success and a model for the necessity of experiencing guilt about having enough money or talent.

A single-parent patient of mine was able to celebrate her son's triumph in unusual circumstances. On the afternoon of the session Meg came late, rolling in drunk with Kevin, a new friend who had been persuaded to drive her to the session. Meg sat at once behind the instruments and asked if Kevin could stay. I agreed. (He was not drunk). Meg said that she had never told me that she was alcoholic. She had drunk eight bottles of wine during the weekend and another bottle and some liqueur that day. She kept saying that she was dying for a drink. We explored this feeling and what it was that she really wanted and she thought it was love. We talked about a baby getting love and drink together, if all was well. Suddenly she sat looking as if she might cry, and I mentioned this. Yes, she did feel like crying. I asked about the parents' coffee morning to which she had said she had been invited . Yes, it was great, they all liked her; then suddenly she remembered that she had seen the teacher of her son Nigel. "He's top of the class," she shouted almost unable to believe it. "The only child in the class who can READ," her voice rose to a squeak. Since she had realised her sadness she had not mentioned drink. I said, "Shall we celebrate Nigel's reading?" She agreed: "But I've no whiskey so we'll have to use music." Kevin was given a Cuban drum to play but not from Meg's own battery of instruments.

Before we began Meg forgot what we were celebrating. Was it envy or alcohol that had snatched it away? I reminded her and she was enthusiastic. Her music was quite different from the delicate baby music she played when sober. She banged down on the xylophone with both beaters in rhythmic moderato crotchets, the wooden notes clacking as they bounced and jumped off the instrument. Kevin played a gentle, accompanying drumming. He seemed an unusually sensitive and adaptable person; and he in no way interfered with the therapy. When we heard the tape back Meg said how, when she was pregnant, she had patted her tummy and said "You shall have everything that I never had." She had been very deprived. "It must make you quite envious of him," I said, but she was not ready to face this yet.

Somehow Meg had felt that she was not allowed to be the mother of the most successful boy in the class until the event was distinguished by our musical ceremony. It became a fact which was accepted and celebrated by a representative nucleus of the community.

Taken at its most primitive level, lack of celebration can be equated with the mother who takes the full pot and flushes the infant's faeces away without comment or interest. An internalised mother of this kind could make life endlessly grey without any high points or festivals of gratitude and delight. Happy events would go unrewarded and all would boil down to a uniform grey sludge. For men have always needed their celebrations; they have lived and died and left little else behind them. Stones on hilltops, strange buildings and sculptures, great musical structures, solemn religious rites, and shapes of lovely dances all point to the lives of those who dared to celebrate, and dared to be enviable.

The event which has not been celebrated seems to be something that you cannot build on; it is not a valid step on the ladder; it has not been accepted by a representative of the community as in an initiation rite, and is therefore open to being swept away by envious attacks and destruction both from within and without. Also eroding, but often well-meant, is the instant pointing to a further goal, instead of celebrating the present achievement and allowing some refuelling time before a new supply of energy and enthusiasm has developed.

Sometimes the celebration of an acquisition can lead the patient to a deeper valuation of herself as an acquisition of her parents. Greta was a separated teacher of thirty who came to her session in rather a muddled mood; there seemed to be some confusion between mothering and being mothered. She had bought and was delighted with a new, brilliant green car, and had stripped and painted some chairs at home. She told me that she was standing by to step in and look after her sister-in-law's children when their mother went into hospital to have her baby. Greta said that she decided not to have a baby herself while she was without a husband. We had discussed this in another session and she said that she thought that I must feel very strongly about it to have given my opinion, which wrongly or rightly, I did.

She remembered her father pushing food into her when she was in her high chair and how she vomited and was put in her room. I wondered if this was a warning about the opinion which she may have felt was forced into her by me. At the end of the session we reached back to the green car and the painted chairs to celebrate. She played xylophone quavers with chaotic excitement then her music was jaunty and affirmative. Afterwards she said she felt her mother tucking her up in bed. This was a typical very early sensation-type flashback memory which patients can experience in a very healing way in this kind of therapy, and it was quite a step for Greta to allow herself to feel mothered.

Then she asked if I would come to supper with her, immediately wanting to regain the nurturing role. I didn't want to come but thanked her for the invitation and we went out briefly together to admire the green car.

Not every patient is able or willing to celebrate, and the therapist will be sensitive enough not to push a patient beyond what she feels able to do. As said earlier, for some the act of celebration is felt to arouse such a threatening level of envy in others that to carry it out would evoke unmanageable persecutory anxiety. A celebration should really be a generous and trusting act of gratitude, a sharing of happiness with others who are felt to be loving enough to enjoy this. But, as Melanie Klein (1975) wrote: "The fact that envy spoils the capacity for enjoyment explains to some extent why envy is so persistent. For it is enjoyment and the gratitude to which it gives rise that mitigate destructive impulses, envy and greed."

Of course all this creates a vicious circle. The envied hides away from the envier for fear of the evil eye in one form or another, and thus the envier cannot be shown what steps need to be taken to acquire such an envied possession, creation, relationship or occupation ---or even to share one with the envied owner. Thus the envier cannot discover his own inner wealth gained by whatever strengths of his own he may have. He cannot see his way to being a creator so becomes a destroyer.

Sometimes a celebration misfires in that it evokes not joy but just those persecutors, often from within, which have been feared. Nora, a manic-depressive patient, came to a session on her fortieth birthday. She talked about the relationships in her office for some time and said that her boss had said that he thought she had progressed well during the last eighteen months especially with eye contact and the ability to hold a conversation. (It was striking that she had manipulated him into assessing her as a patient rather than as a worker at her desk job in his office). She could not give our therapy a direct compliment but felt safer speaking through him. We decided to play about her fortieth birthday. It could have been an opportunity for celebration but her music was tentative, jerky and anxious. She felt angry because jobs stopped being offered at forty, clubs closed their doors to the forties and there was less chance, she thought, of getting married. Although there was a certain amount of truth in her statements, I felt that she was enviously spoiling her remaining days and denying that there was anything at all to celebrate in the first forty years. It was not an encouraging pattern.

Affirmations are somewhat different from celebrations, they represent musically a positive declaration about a happening. Small children demand them continually: "Wasn't that a lovely rainbow we saw in the park today?" or "Can't I run fast?" or "Isn't my white mouse handsome?". Verbally an analytical music therapist will avoid them as it is not his intention to make the patient as dependent on him as she was on her mother. But musically, that is another matter. To demand assurance from the therapist and to get it, is not the same as going back to an important moment in time and space and oneself recreating the feeling about it in sound, and then sharing this experience with the therapist. In the latter the assurance and affirmation come from within the patient; she is seeking her own strength and offering to share her delight in it with the therapist and not, as in the former, weakly depending on him for strength and affirmation. Affirmations usually come about when the patient has been in therapy for some time and feels comfortable enough to reach back in her mind and find something splendid that she wants to share. That is the moment to make a musical affirmation.

Dennis, a man in his thirties, was recalling a time in his teens when he and a friend had gone spear-fishing in the sea. He played music describing his feelings about this absorbing time, long before any signs of his schizophrenic illness. He played in regular but spikey quavers on the xylophone with occasional significant changes in tempo. He recalled fishing in the wrong place for a whole year before a fisherman showed him the rocks near where the fish lay in the sand. He would breathe deeply, dive down and spear the fish and hook them on to a ring on his belt. Once home, his grandfather would help to clean them and his mother would cook them. Sometimes his father, on his way to work, would see Dennis swimming out to spear the fish, and wave. While Dennis told me this with much pleasure in his memories and my interest in them, he held the two beaters together at an angle of 45 degrees from the top of his thigh like a mock erection. It was surely a time when he had felt his growing manhood strongly and satisfyingly used in this symbolic way and our playing together affirmed this.

Quite often the happening affirmed evokes qualities that have somehow been forgotten along the way. The patient indeed seems to be fishing something out and saying: "Look, I've got this and I had quite forgotten that I ever had it!" Dennis had not been able to live a particularly virile life since his illness and this experience that we shared was a regained treasure.

Some weeks before, we had seen another aspect of this. In this session I was saying to Dennis that he created a gentle peaceful world for himself and me, and kept everything bad outside. He agreed that he did this, he did not like quarrels or all the violence on television. But then he spoke up for himself. At school, he said, he did once defend his friend Sam against the whole form. The other children in his form were chanting taunts at Sam and bullying him physically when Dennis stepped in, rescued him and became his friend. We decided to affirm this with an improvisation called "Standing up for Sam." The bullying was played in triplets on the drum, it was quite fierce. Then came a reiterated minor upward-going phrase on the xylophone then up and down, more varied with three against four between our parts and ending with a gentle, flowing and more adventurous 6/8 melody. He expressed far more emotion than he usually did and I think felt a proper pride in his action. It was as if he said, "I am also this kind of man."

It is very important to be aware of something of a patient's being throughout the whole line of his life as, following illness, he can be little more in the present than a caricature of his true self. To know something more of his whole self gives him a dignity in his own and his therapist's eyes which contributes greatly to his ability to be healed. It makes me sad to see, and indeed to have personally experienced, in what an undignified way psychiatric patients are often hounded and herded to their meals and medication in institutions as if their present state of apathy and anxiety were the only being they had ever had and their former lives as mothers and grandmothers, teachers, doctors of music and priests were totally irrelevant. But I digress.

The therapist is not able to use every strong image that a patient brings up. Such an image came up with a male patient of thirty-two but as we were in the initial stages of therapy we were working on another line and we did not musically affirm it. However, it was an important memory, no doubt we will come back to it. I will describe it here. Donald was about eight years old and playing in the tall bracken with his dog when suddenly he turned a corner and looked up at a huge stag with spreading antlers which stood over him. The image ended there. No doubt phantasy had blocked off the reality.

However, not all affirmations turn out happily. Barbara was a woman in her fifties having schizophrenia, she had been stitched together tenuously by twenty-two years of psychotherapy. She arrived at this session half an hour late as she had been to an exhibition of butterflies that was very lovely. She chose to play music about the butterflies on the D major diatonic glockenspiel in even 4/4 crotchets. Our music was rather idyllic but as we played there was a counter-transference of sadness which I allowed into the music with some E minor and B minor chords. Barbara left her session with a feeling of disappointment, perhaps because those butterflies had cheated her of half the time we should have had together in the present of here-and-now. Perhaps I should have kept that sadness to myself for the time being. One ponders and questions and learns.

Sometimes one is delightfully surprised with an affirmation. A young man said that he had been noticing the prunus blossom in the next street and wanted to affirm this experience in an improvisation on spring. Somehow, although I myself love the spring, I gave a silent inward groan. I suppose I felt "It has been done to death by Mendelssohn." But he gave me a lovely experience. He used his voice with a smooth richness that I had not heard before and evoked a blissful calm that was extremely beautiful and would have done credit to Faure. Rather than being just his usual musical escape from the unpleasant sides of his life, this music seemed to be full of rich and mysterious possibilities for growth and development. I felt ashamed of my weary distrust of the inspiration of this great period of renewal in nature and our lives.

I left this essay as one of the later ones because our musical celebrations and affirmations are for occasional use. They do not form the bread and butter of analytical music therapy, although psychodynamic understanding may help the therapist to decide on the advisablity of using or not using one in any given session. Nor should they be confused with "Magical Solutions" where the patient hopes omnipotently to influence an external event by playing about it. Of course he can influence his own attitude to it and thereby change a situation, but danger lies in imagining that he, himself, can change it in a godlike way.

Neither should these "Magical Solutions" be confused with "Reality Rehearsals" which can flush out unconscious fears about a forthcoming event so that these can be helped by discovering just what the real fear is in that situation and working on it. These and many other techniques are described in my previous book (Priestley, 1975). Our affirmations are confident assertions that it was indeed so, and our celebrations help our patients to have the courage to stand up and be envied, without needing to resort to manic enviableness. To be able, with Walt Whitman, to say:" I celebrate myself, and sing myself."

Essay Twenty-Two

Case Study Of A Depressed Patient

We in the music therapy department of the psychiatric hospital where I worked for twenty years, felt grateful to have had the opportunity to work with so many different people with almost as many unique kinds of personal damage, though often given the same labels. However, to protect our younger colleagues full of initial zeal and idealism, we have to admit that the work had many frustrating aspects. Patients would often be discharged without our knowledge just as the work looked as if it was getting somewhere. Occasionally a senior colleague from another discipline swooped down and took over a case that was looking quite promising, not always with brilliant results. Sessions could be interrupted in the middle of sensitive interactions by one's patient being called to wash up, or they could be obliviated by the patient being whisked off to a trip to Brighton.

This was, of course, because in our initial zeal and idealism we wanted to pack in as much contact work as possible in our two days there. This meant that we did not always take time to nurture the vital links with other staff. Thus decisions would be made on the days when we were doing work elsewhere with no communication coming through to our department. The result, in my case, was frustration and fury. Present-day colleagues are more aware of the need for establishing interdisciplinary lines of communiciation and links as well as developing their personal work with patients. However, now and then one was able to complete a bit of work and feel quite good about it. This case study was one of those happier occasions, though admittedly this patient was far less damaged than many with whom we worked. As usual all identifying details have been altered or omitted and the name changed.

Lillian came to the psychiatric hospital in April and was referred by her psychiatrist to music therapy in May that year. She joined the patients' choir run by the Head Music Therapist Gillian Lovett, and was the ideal patient: polite, intelligent, thoughtful and musical. However, Gillian thought that she needed more radical treatment and so suggested to the psychiatrist that I should take her on for analytical music therapy.

Lillian, thirty-four, was small and slim, with bushy red hair, a pointed nose and pleasant face lit by her undoubted intelligence. She described herself as "introverted, not a very happy person, I've lost things I used to do, like squash." She was born overseas and had come to this country eight years ago. She had had an extremely taxing and responsible job in a large firm but, becoming depressed, she had accepted a less demanding post working as an assistant to someone who was doing a job similar to the one she had just left. She was depressed but on no medication, and spasmodically attended the hospital psychologist's therapy group as well as the choir.

On the day of her first session (my first in the morning), the buses were held up and I was twenty minutes late. She was waiting. I took her history. She couldn't speak to her mother. Her father was "remote," and she did not get on with an elder sister. She thought that her trouble was that because of difficulties in her private life she had pushed herself to work harder and harder at her job. She had been ambitious and thought that having a good job was everything, but she now felt that being happy was more important. I pointed out that these aims were not necessarily mutually exclusive.

Her immediate problem was that her television needed a new aerial and she had told the man to come between 4:00 and 5:00 PM. He had come before that, when she was still in hospital, and left a card to say he had found no one in. She felt really furious with him for being so inefficient in his job when there was all this unemployment, but felt that she could not confront him. I said she must have been equally angry with me being late this morning. "Oh no!" and so on.

I took for our improvisation title "Telling the Aerial Man". She held the beaters and erupted into great convulsive sobs. I shouted "Put it into action" and with a moan she crashed down on the cymbal and pounded fiercely on the drum. Then she cried again. Once more I asked her to put that into action and she drummed furiously and then played some glissandi to soothe herself. When she finished, smiling and tearful, she said that she had thought that music therapy was listening to music on records to soothe herself, like she did at home.

Next week she returned, looking much firmer, brighter and less guilty. She had seen the aerial man and told him what she thought. She had taken something back to a shop, and played squash, even scoring (which she previously had not been able to do). She said that she had a "thing" about knives so we used "Knives" as a title, but her music was less explosive and her thoughts were of the rejecting and accepting aspects of her family, and thoughts about her job prospects. I said that she had not been using her aggression assertively until recently and she had projected it outside and symbolised it as threatening knives or frightening split-off possibilities of using aggression.

Next week she spoke about meeting a young man with her girl friend and freezing him out, so the girlfriend grabbed him. She played her feelings about this with great energy but no longer wept.

Next week she faced discharge from the hospital and I offered to see her at 6:00 PM as an outpatient. She agreed to this. It was the end of choir. The man had not rung her. She felt boring. We played "Ringing Ken." There was panic and anger at being put in this situation then she remembered, to gentle music, how nice he was. She never imagined speaking to him. I said I thought that she was angry with me for putting her in this situation. "Oh no, neutral with staff," she replied. Then we played "Telling Ken What I Think of Him," using angry clashes followed by sweet, docile music.

Next week she said that she had rung Ken and he was coming to supper, bringing tomato soup. She had refused a more taxing job at work. She kept mentioning "Being Dull" so we took this for a title. Her music was discordant and lively, then aggressive and empty, and I said it was punishing my delicate and plaintive melodies. She was not ready to see this. She felt that dullness covered all these fierce feelings that she was now using. I said she was afraid of what she might do as she had, as she had said, been a tag-along friend and was unused to initiating events.

At the next session she reported a set-back all round. At work she had been put on the pay-roll and given no job. Ken had brought the soup but had been bent on sex, which she did not feel ready for, and she had had to throw him out. A dominant girlfriend, Zoe, had invited her to a raspberry supper party that lasted for hours, ending up in a nightclub at 3:00 AM. Every time she had wanted to leave, Zoe said "Don't be so boring." She felt suicidal when she got home. We played "Zoe," to get back her projection on to this friend, and her music was direct and aggressive.

Next week I was ill and had to miss the session. The week after, Lillian was exploring the reason why she had not told her parents about her illness. We played "Telling Parents." She didn't want to write, was angry with herself, got blocked and ended up dreaming of a really free communication. She was very angry with her parents for sweeping family secrets under the carpet: a breakdown here, an illegitimacy there, an odd in-law, and so on.

Next week, the last of the two first months, she was back at work, in total chaos, with no desk, and not taking her lunch hour. She wondered how much unreasonableness was hers and how much was theirs. She decided to have lunch every day, stick to two early nights, and create her own small territory at work. I did not record the music in my journal.

As a result of the session before, she did write to her parents and had a loving telegram by return from her mother. She organised her office and sorted out that she was to have only one boss.

By the tenth session she was quite rid of her depression and the aggression was directed outwards: she was in a foul temper and expressed this dynamically on the drum and cymbal. By the fourteenth session she said she felt so good that she wanted to stop. It transpired that she feared dependency. She was brought up to be independent but had a secret longing, of which she was ashamed, to lean on someone. I was experiencing countertransference feelings of acute inadequacy, and told her that she still had these feelings to explore. She said she had always felt a failure and so had run away. Her flight to England was part of this pattern.

In the sixteenth session she reported that she was really happy, having held a good and adventurous dinner party. She had been high the week before but this was real solid happiness. The celebrating music was quite dizzy and fun. She gave up the group therapy.

In the twentieth session she said she had been assertive in the office but was afraid of being irrational. Her imagination exercise about an irritating colleague, Lena, revealed Lillian cutting off Lena's head, chopping her to bits and throwing them in to the sea to be eaten by lions. By talion law she feared "losing her head" and being "cut up." She laughed uproariously when I pointed this out. (This is not an exercise for psychotic patients).

In the twenty-second session she said her married friends who had met through a marriage bureau asked why she didn't try this. She wanted to do so and I agreed to extend the session until Easter.

In the four last sessions she struggled with her feelings of inadequacy, and met two unsuitable men. Work went well and she was more alive but more vulnerable to anxiety. In her last session she realised that either she would have to change her old social patterns now or she would end up like her maiden aunt, Kathy, solitary and embittered. She also realised that music therapy was not a magic wand and she, herself, would have to do the work. She was rather apprehensive about stopping and we agreed on a four-month follow-up.

At the follow-up she looked well but a bit defended. She had had some depressive happenings but had been able to sort them out for herself without getting depressed. She had met three men, discarded two and kept one as a friend with whom she planned to do some clothes designing. Work was boring but she did not want to take on a more responsible position. She had been bad about keeping up with friends, as she had been seeing a lot of her neighbour. Evidently she thought that this was a depressing note to end on, so sent me a card saying: "I wanted to let you know how grateful I am to you for your help and quiet confidence-building over the last year. I have appreciated beyond words the help everyone at the hospital has given me, but particularly the patience and care you have shown me. I cannot thank you enough but I hope you know how much it has all meant to me. Thank you for everything."

What did the music mean to her? I think finding an outlet for her aggression in a harmless way gave her the courage to use it assertively in life situations. I think that it also gave her the power to face her own painful feelings of inadequacy in the containing dyadic improvisations and then explore these in words. She was a fighter and in many ways a delightful patient, but struggling with the countertransference inadequacy feelings before she was ready to face them herself was very uncomfortable for the therapist. In a way the therapy was painful for her too, as she exchanged her global depression for an awareness of all that she needed to do to create a satisfying life for herself. The therapy did not end with a magical solution to all her problems but rather presented her with a possible new beginning, which she sadly lacked at the start of the work.

Essay Twenty-Three

Music And The Shadow

All therapists seek to help their client's change in some way. Jungian therapy places a premium on understanding the patient and the patient's strengths, weaknesses, and needs, both conscious and unconscious. Central to Jungian theory is the concept of the shadow, or personal unconscious, that region of the mind which contains lost memories, impulses, instincts, and ideas which are not acceptable to the ego-consciousness and are therefore repressed.

A deeper region containing archaic, archetypal, and instinctive inheritances Jung called the collective unconscious. Its contents are neither repressed nor available to normal consciousness. Jung (1958) said, however, that they can be dragged into consciousness when one works with the shadow (Volume 12, p. 32). "There (in the collective unconscious) I am utterly one with the world, so much part of it that I forget all too easily who I really am" (Jung, 1958, Volume 9, p. 22).

When the shadow is not acknowledged, a person either rejects it totally and becomes a flat, shallow personality, or s/he projects its contents onto others, disapproving of them violently. Many people reject their shadows because, "We do not like to look at the shadow side of ourselves, therefore there are many people in our civilized society who have lost their shadow altogether, they have got rid of it. They are only two-dimensional, they have lost their third dimension and with it they have usually lost the body" (Jung, 1958, Volume 18, p. 23).

When a person projects his/her shadow, baser instincts and suppressed envy, jealousy, and greed are only seen in others. Jung (1958, Volume 11, p. 83) wrote: "We must still be exceedingly careful not to project our own shadow too shamelessly, we are still swamped with projected illusions. If you imagine someone who is brave enough to withdraw all these projections, then you get an individual who is conscious of a pretty thick shadow. Such a man has saddled himself with new problems and conflicts."

Jung (1958, Volume 9 [II], p. 8) wrote the following: "The shadow is a moral problem that challenges the whole ego-personality, for no one can become conscious of the shadow without considerable moral effort. To become conscious of it involves recognizing the dark aspects of the personality as present and real. This act is the essential condition for any kind of self-knowledge, and it therefore, as a rule, meets with considerable resistance. Indeed, self-knowledge as a psycho-therapeutic measure frequently requires much painstaking work extended over a long period."

Knowing one's shadow requires working with another person and is the first step in any thorough personal analysis. Intellectual knowledge about the shadow is, if anything, only a beginning. "In dealing with the shadow or anima it is not sufficient to know about these concepts and to reflect on them. Nor can we ever experience their content by feeling our way into them or by appropriating other people's feelings" (Jung, 1958, Volume 9 [I], p. 30).

Although knowing one's shadow is not easy and is sometimes frightening, "the shadow and the opposing will are the necessary conditions for all actualizing" (Jung, 1958, Volume 11, p. 196). Action without realization of the shadow is subject to sudden unconscious reversal. Action produced by the tension of opposites can signify true progress. In The Development of Personality, Jung (1958) wrote: "All consciousness, perhaps without being aware of it, seeks its unconscious opposite, lacking which it is doomed to stagnation, congestion and ossification. Life is born only of the spark of the opposites" (p. 53).

It is interesting and important to be aware of Jung's framework when he developed his concept of the shadow. At that point in his career, he had left the Burgholzli Asylum in Zurich. Most of his private patients were not psychotic, but functioning people who felt that they had missed something in their lives. Many of them were in the second half of life. The exploration of this dark shadow was an essential aspect of their discoveries of their whole selves.

Many of the people I treat with music therapy, in contrast, are people who have not fulfilled their potential in even the most basic tasks of life. For them, the shadow also contains hints of unrealized possibilities. Modern Jungians talk about this as the "bright shadow." Jung himself did not directly refer to it as such.

In Aion Jung (1958) wrote: "If it has been believed hitherto that the human shadow was the source of all evil, it can now be ascertained on closer investigation that the unconscious man, that is, his shadow, does not consist only of morally reprehensible tendencies, but also displays a number of good qualities, such as normal instincts, appropriate reactions, realistic insights, creative impulses, etc. On this level evil appears more as a distortion, a deformation, a disinterpretation and misapplication of facts that in themselves are natural" (p. 266).

The potentially good qualities are somehow hidden in the shadow, guarded by impulses which can be all the more dangerous for being unknown. "It is not only the shadow-side that is overlooked, disregarded and repressed; positive qualities can also be subjected to the same treatment" (Jung, 1958, Volume 18, p. 221).

Working with the shadow offers possibilities of healing (in the sense of making whole) and renewing life. Music can be a bridge between consciousness and both the personal and later the collective unconscious. Since music involves instant physical expression, the emotions realized can facilitate insights by making defensiveness more difficult. Jung wrote of the importance of experiencing one's unconscious. "A running commentary is absolutely necessary in dealing with the shadow, because otherwise its actuality cannot be fixed. Only in this painful way is it possible to gain a positive insight into the complex nature of one's own personality" (Jung, 1958, Volume 14, p. 496). Improvised music can provide the immediate link in a directly emotional language, which can afterwards be interpreted with more reflection, in words.

The following case studies show four of my patients who realized the possibility of their potentials for development by experiencing musically an aspect of their shadows.

Case Study: O.B.

O.B.'s piano playing is a good example of the bright shadow, since it is energetic and full of hope and joy. That the music is joyous is at first surprising, because it was composed by a person who was quite depressed, struggling inwardly with suicidal tendencies and outwardly with an extremely difficult job as teacher of aggressive, maladjusted boys. He spent his friendless leisure hours sleeping a great deal. He had severe relationship problems with his aging parents, who lived out of town.

To me, O.B.'s piano playing, whether of composed music or improvisations, has the quality of a seed. The playing seems packed with potential for development, with a tension that longs to expand. I have not experienced any other client with such a seed quality in his playing.

O.B. was a single man in his mid-forties. He was brought up in a household of many women and a father who was often physically or emotionally absent. His powerful relationship with his mother found expression in his early aptitude for the piano. During early adolescence his attitude toward his mother and his music became rejecting. O.B. remained narcissistically stuck at the same stage of adolescence as the boys he teaches. He began therapy after a long history of self-destruction which endangered all aspects of his life, including his capacity to use his remarkable musical gifts. We pursued individual music therapy, focusing on his particular gifts, at the same time as group analytic and individual psychotherapy.

Interestingly, O.B.'s improvised music on percussion, with me at the piano, expressed only his present conflicts, with no joy or hope. When improvising the destructive aspect of his mother, his music was first frenzied and confused, then lost and feeble, and, finally, with a sinister accompaniment on the drum, physically destructive, scattering the loose xylophone notes over the working area. This improvisation sent cold shivers down my back. I try to contain this destruction in major chords and his music ends in sobbing chaos.

O.B.'s improvisations on percussion instruments were explorations of conscious situations, expressing his feelings through the creative medium of our duet music and the discussions that followed. His piano playing, with its seed quality, exhibited a different aspect of O.B. It seemed to be a communication from a totally unknown part of him, equally strange to both of us. It was a message from his shadow, a message even more important than the hopeless, angry drum playing.

Case Study: Z.O.

Z.O. was a married man of sixty-two with children and grandchildren. He had high blood pressure, was tense and agitated, and scarcely spoke. I included him in my Movement, Relaxation, and Communication Therapy Group. Further, he entered individual music therapy because he had the expression of a desperately sad six-month old baby who wanted to be picked up. I couldn't resist it. I picked him up.

From the beginning his improvised music contradicted everything else about him. It was dynamic and confident, and though he said he never had any dreams, his imagination exercises were powerful and vivid.

Like most analytical music therapists, I began our sessions with discussion. The theme that emerges during this period is used as a title for our improvisation. I play the piano and the patient plays on tuned and untuned percussion instruments. After our music there is more talk.

Z.O.'s improvised music was an expression of his bright shadow, a dynamism evident nowhere else in his life. Our work gradually convinced him that this creativity was a vital part of himself. It was raging at his redundancy, his inability to keep up with his peers financially, and his envy of his wife's enjoyment of her amateur hobbies. It demanded life. He had to take the responsibility for these feelings as well as his more acceptable positive ones.

At the beginning of his music therapy, he spent much time lying in bed at home. He dreaded talking to people he didn't know, thinking he had nothing to say and feeling inferior because he had no job and little money. After one year's therapy, Z.O. had an apparent setback, undergoing a period of regressive behavior. He was admitted to the hospital when he refused to shave or dress and even became temporarily incontinent. When I saw him on the ward, we shared our mutual helplessness. His music had convinced me, however, that behind this wish to be a baby, and cared for totally, was a search for wholeness. After four months, he returned home, continuing to come once weekly to music therapy and biweekly to the Music, Relaxation and Communication Therapy Group. By his second year, his blood pressure was normal.

During his third year of therapy, improvisational music played an important part in his communication and growth. For example, the week before a particular session, I reminded him that we had agreed that he should begin to come monthly at the end of that month. This time he announced rather triumphantly that he had not been pleased with himself. His wife, screaming and shouting, had had to pull him out of bed. I interpreted that he was feeling abandoned by me as he had been by his mother who had died when he was a boy, and he wanted to curl up and be a baby. "Being Abandoned" was the title of his improvisation. His statement on the xylophone was almost indignant. Then his trill expressed anxiety and the drums anger, but he felt that he could and would cope.

After another year of music therapy he had gained in confidence. He coped with visitors and strangers, played with his grandchildren, helped to care for disabled people on a voluntary basis, and could navigate for his driving wife. His fear of getting physically lost prevented him from taking the wheel himself, but it wasn't the panic it used to be.

Z.O.'s consultant psychiatrist, Dr. Lewis, was so impressed with Z.O.'s progress that he wrote: "I have seldom seen a patient with such a high degree of chronicity and almost despaired of seeing him well again---or even significantly improved. Over the past eighteen months or so, however, he has shown signs of considerable and dramatic improvement. This impression would appear to be the result of intervention by the Music Therapist and is a significant and dramatic example of what can be achieved by Music Therapy."

If Z.O.'s music had not shown such vitality, I might have considered him hopeless when he was admitted. His music, however, had revealed his shadow to me---a part of him that was seeking an outlet in life. It was an as yet unrealized part of his being. At that time, I was the only one on the therapeutic team who believed he could progress. But only I had heard his music.

Case Study: S.R.

Music can express many sides of the personality. The music of S.R., an almost mute schizophrenic youth of 18, expressed first a gentle, almost secret rhythmic sensitivity, then a rigid rhythm on untuned percussion. He allowed himself so little body awareness that he would have continued with one rhythm and instrument for 50 minutes if I had let him. After several sessions a feeling of insecurity and distrust of relationships was expressed in an unsteady pulse which somehow always avoided my accompaniment. In later sessions came a feeling of self-affirmation with a full, steady beat, allowing increasing body awareness.

Over a period of four months came a marked increase in verbal communication and facial expression in therapy sessions. At home his father reported greater tolerance of body contact, greater cheerfulness and socialization, a quite regressive demand for affection by cuddling and holding, and a surprising walk alone to the library to get books on his favorite subjects.

S.R.'s most important impulse from the shadow exhibited itself not in instrumental music but in body music. One day during therapy I decided to just sit silently: do nothing but just be with him. As I sat, my mind wandered. He suddenly gave me a piercing look and clapped his hands. I was jerked into awareness and clapped back. He clapped. I clapped. As the clapping continued, his face was alive and wreathed in smiles. In the ensuing Music, Relaxation and Communication group sessions he would clap and I would respond whenever he felt that he was being overlooked. It was his greeting in the morning and his demand for affirmation that he did exist and that his feelings mattered to me. It was a much more spontaneous and expressive communication than either his halting, stilted words or his autistic-sounding improvised music. Most importantly, it was his original creation. Without using words, S.R. was able to retrieve from his shadow the long-lost impulse to spontaneously express his longing for a relationship to someone who mattered to him.

Case Study: B.L.

My final example, B.L., was 55, single, a second-generation white Russian, bearded, toothless, and of enormous size. He was referred to me by an art therapist. His singing voice was penetrating and powerful. At the beginning of our nine months in individual sessions he was manic: roaring his anger, clashing the cymbals and banging the drum, and singing Russian and Polish songs in bursts of enthusiasm. Reality, with his now frail and elderly father (who had formerly been the stable centre of his life) and his girlfriend, who herself had frequent breakdowns, was not something that he wished to explore. He shared with me his eventful and happy childhood overseas. It was the best part of his life and in some ways he had never left it. His mother died when he was 19 years old and he had his first breakdown some months afterwards. His total lack of grief work---he played volleyball on the day of the funeral---may have contributed to his first paranoid psychotic episode.

For nine months in music therapy his improvised music mirrored his wildest escapist stance, but as the months went by he became quieter, more thoughtful, and more depressed. He awoke dreading each day, but was more and more able to tolerate examining his external reality and even to wonder what he would do after the death of his father.

Speaking of his relationship with his father and his girlfriend, he expressed irritation, "Bloody Hell! I have to do this for her and that for him." I asked him what it was he really wanted to do since he felt so irritated by the work that these two relationships entailed. He didn't know. He had never known. We entitled the next improvisation "What I Want To Do." Something totally surprising to both of us emerged. His xylophone playing was weak and indecisive in a childlike treble sound pattern. When I commented that it had never been like that before, he burst out, "That is me. I am really like that inside. I pretend to be so strong with my great voice singing and shouting and smashing windows but really I am very weak." This vulnerability was his unrealized potential, long hidden in his shadow and overlaid by manic behaviour.

At this point, B.L. revealed that he was having suicidal

thoughts. Overdosing had been his habitual response to stress in the past. As he was an out-patient and not under the care of a psychiatrist, I contacted his doctor, suggesting that he be referred for extra help during this difficult period. Before help could be obtained, he was overcome by his shadow, impulsively combining whiskey with all his pills. Luckily, as he was such a large man, he awoke the next morning, apparently unharmed. He had no memory of buying the whiskey, showing that his was an identification with the shadow rather than a deliberate conscious action.

B.L.'s improvisation had indicated that he wanted to relate to others from his vulnerability, rather than always defending it by his manic behaviour. He needed to know this part of his shadow and accept it instead of letting himself be overcome by it. Our music revealed his shadowed weakness which held the potential of his true strength and further development.

Conclusion

Music can express any emotion, conscious or unconscious. It can be the brittle music of defense, the shallow passing mood of the moment or a hauntingly deep voice from the shadow which may need a great deal of therapy before it is safely assimilated into the patient's consciousness. It takes training and experience to be aware of the seminal nature of these musical suggestions from the shadow, but when they are answered at the right moment and in the right way, radical healing can take place. Jung (1958, Volume 9 [I]. p. 291) himself said: "In the case of the individual, the problem constellated by the shadow is answered on the plane of the anima, that is, through relatedness. In the history of the collective as in the history of the individual, everything depends on the development of the consciousness, This gradually brings liberation from imprisonment in ayvoia (unconsciousness) and is therefore a bringer of light as well as of healing."

Essay Twenty-Four

Music And The Listeners

This essay outlines fourteen sessions of analytical music therapy spread over six months and a follow-up session thirteen weeks later. The client, Renata, was a self-referred lady psychotherapist aged 60. She had one isolated problem which many sessions of psychotherapy had failed to touch, so in fact this was a focal music therapy. Her problem was that she could not play, or even practice the piano, if she felt anyone (including her teacher) was listening. If she did, she had feelings of panic and had to stop. This reduced her playing to the very minimum and naturally hindered her progress and her enjoyment of this art. As she was approaching a more leisured time of life she felt that it was now crucial to try and overcome this anxiety.

This essay is based on brief notes made after sessions and a re-hearing of the recorded improvisations. The client's name and some circumstances have been concealed to preserve confidentiality. She has seen the case study and given her permission to publish. In order to give the feeling of the inner meaning and emotional flavour of an utterance, words or sentences in quotes are the client's own. Discussion recorded before the improvisation took place before we played. The supervisor mentioned twice is the Jungian analyst, Dr. Redfearn, with whom the writer has discussed her work for several years. The 50-minute sessions were weekly as far as possible, but dates are given.

3/2/86. As I have found so often with female clients with performing difficulties, it came out in the anamnesis that Renata's music had come from her father, who had played the piano. There also had been chamber music in the home. Her early life was quite difficult. She had a Down's Syndrome sister Anna, 15 months older than her, whom she sensitively watched over until Anna's death when Renata was 7 years old. When visitors came, Anna was always introduced first and Renata felt almost ashamed of her own greater accomplishments and remembered being refused a bicycle as Anna could not cope with one. When Renata was 5 1/2, another sister, Kate, was born.

I asked Renata to play in the role of "The Listeners" hoping that she might get back her projections of punitive and critical self-parts. The improvisation (which I accompanied on the piano) was short but full of character. She wept. She felt that her left hand was clumsy, letting down the piece. We played "Left Hand" which was very sensitive and beautiful with what she called a "murderous" ugly, banging right hand. I said it was sounding very bossy. She said: "The right hand said 'Don't do that!' and then turned it into not music at all, while the left hand was like making love using fingers on the keys."

10/2/86. She said that she thought her teacher was coming back in three weeks and she had started to make mistakes. I said she could allow herself to need him, but I did not realise at this point that it was for the purpose of self-punishment. She said that he insisted that she couldn't play in front of him because of her lack of practice. She remembered that Anna was always praised if she had a dry bed but Renata's was taken for granted. Kate had temper tantrums at 3. Renata envied her freedom but thought: "That is not in my repertoire." Renata had never had a temper tantrum in her life. She had been the observing, caring child, then the doctor doing research, then the psychiatrist, then had psychotherapy and practised as a psychotherapist. She was almost retired but felt the need to do something completely different.

She played as the "Carer" while I played as "Temper Tantrums." Hearing me, she felt panicky and played the bells as she felt there was some emergency. Her xylophone playing was gentle and the bells were soft. I felt I could not let go when playing as the "Temper Tantrums," as I felt she couldn't tolerate really wild playing at that point. We exchanged roles. Her "Temper Tantrums" sounded demanding and assertive as if she was saying "Look at ME!" Later it was sad and childlike with the odd bang in between. She managed to split the drumhead, prolong the session by five minutes and forget to pay me.

17/2/86. She felt that our improvisation last time had not been so musical. I said that temper tantrums are not very musical. I suggested that we examine the feelings about not paying. "Not worth it comes to mind," she replied sharply. I pointed out that it can also mean that the relationship is being regarded as a friendly one rather than a professional one. She said that she hadn't thought of that. She felt "a bit embarrassed at not having paid, but not very." She had improvised at home and thought she would feel less anxious if she was overheard doing that. She said practice was joyless. I wondered whether this was a defence against too much joy but admitted that there were plateaus in all instrumental learning. My supervisor had suggested that we explore last week's "Something Completely Different" (see 10/2/86 session). I asked her to imagine a long, high wall with these words on the door and to go through the door (See Assagioli, 1968). She approached the door twice then went through in the dark and quickly rushed round trying to look at the packing cases which were there. I said there could have been curiosity about mother's part in producing little Kate. She played the kalimba gently then there were knockings and shakings of maracas. I said "Go in again but take your time." She did so and said there was no need of light. She felt that she was being responded to.

The music was freely expressive with xylophone glissandi and maracas, drum taps and two taps on the edge of the xylophone, feeling "Can nasty feelings be accepted too?" She wept. I asked if she cried because she felt understood. "No. Just responded to," she replied.

24/2/86. In the past week, sometimes she had felt like a child and sometimes like a competent adult therapist. Her piano practice went badly and she kept making mistakes. I said this seems to have a persecutory feeling about it. "Yes," she replied. I said she didn't seem to be allowed to be playful and expressive. She played to the title "Mother." The overblown recorder sounded frantic with long melodica notes in between, then came a gentle, carefully played xylophone melody finishing with a long melodica tone. She said she was desperately wanting loving attention. "Mother had been a cold, intelligent person." The concordant identification was of sadness. Next we played "Father." The burst of colourful and expressive music was quite joyful with several instruments played in a confident rhythm. Later it sounded more secretive as if she must hide this. She said that she could have fun with her father in a way that Anna couldn't and she felt guilty about this. Underneath she had really hated Anna and was glad that she died when Renata was seven but had missed her as her personal "job," as she felt it her duty to take care of her. As a young person, a war baby, she felt grey and shapeless but at teenage she felt that her father liked her better than her mother. I said that in her "Father" music there was everything that seemed to be missing in her practice. She said that it was more difficult for her to express tenderness than anger. When I said "Time," she said "It is 5 past." (She came at 2:15, and my sessions last 50 minutes). I pointed this out and she said "Oh, yes."

17/3/86. She felt very limp after influenza and hadn't played. She thought maybe she should have cancelled the forthcoming course that she was giving abroad. She had seen her clients for half of last week. She sat silent then suggested that we should play some limp music. I pulled out the box of chime bars. She played in a slow 4/4 but gradually it became more lively and assertive. I said the music was going ahead to tell us about liveliness. Next we played about "The Course." The music was very direct and confident and multi-instrumental as in the "Father" music. She felt "I'll show you I can do it though I've had flu." I felt it sounded quite petulant and then confident. I said the music represented a very intimate phantasy relationship with her father that went way back and that it explained the guilt when she was discovered playing. She agreed. However, I said, it was now necessary for her to de-sensitise herself to this situation by playing to people. She felt she should be "right" by 60 but felt that the work was worthwhile. I asked her how old her eldest client was. She told me: "60." She said she did not feel hopeful on the way here but now felt better and would like another 5 to 10 sessions.

7/4/86. We played "Stealing Father." She played grasping, grabbing, triumphant piano music to my drum and cymbal. In "Renata, Father and Kate" she played treble and low bass up and down the piano with a chaotic quarrelling sound, followed by a monotone tune interrupted by chords. Lastly, we improvised on "Playing." She explored single note and clusters on the piano finishing with a megacluster.

14/4/86. She cancelled but told me that she had managed to play to her sister Kate.

21/4/86. We decided to explore the feelings about "Right" and "Wrong." To her, "Right" meant right feeling and phrasing and "Wrong" meant it was wrong to play at all. "Right" (on instruments) sounded wooden and priggish on the melodica, then rebellious. "Wrong" started with her coming in very expressively on the xylophone and the whole piece seemed to disintegrate into dissonant xylophone tone clusters and come to a halt. "Wrong" (on piano) she held one hand with the other and played with it as if it were a tool, then she took off her red shoes and played with the tips of her toes. The "Wrong" felt right and she was all alight and glowing with creativity. I then asked her to play her easy pieces on the piano while I took the role of her harsh "Super-ego" saying "Wrong!" and so on. Maybe I went too far when I said "Silly cow! She's done it again!" I hoped that she would build up some resistance against this critical self-part. She persevered in her playing but her concentration seemed to disintegrate and she felt like crying. I wondered if I had overdone it. As it happened, I had.

12/5/86. She hadn't practised and she wanted to stop the sessions. I agreed but said she was like a person who had been clamped in one position for years. When the clamps were removed with difficulty, unless she moved she might as well not have bothered. I emphasised that now it was up to her to test reality by playing to people and seeing that no harm would come to her. At last she said perhaps she would come for a few more sessions and that possibly she had been influenced by the last session. My supervisor had suggested letting her be the Super-ego. We tried this. She shouted sarcastically at me that I was showing off, it was too wooden, there was too much pedal and so on. In fact, it gave me quite a shock too. (I seldom try a technique on a client that I have not tried on myself with one of my colleagues, but I had reacted quite spontaneously to the situation last week. However, it is a rule that I recommend to other music therapists. One can see what happened when I ignored it). Next we improvised "Playing Like Anna." The playing was much more spontaneous and rather angry. We did "Playing II." We played well together like chamber music (no recording and my notes didn't say on what instruments). She decided to play duets and do improvisations with her "cellist friend at home."

19/5/86. She actually had played to a friend. It was very dead. Then she improvised a little and her friend liked it. She was seeing the notes as a mould killing her creativity. We did "Deadness to Life:" she started playing one of her pieces in a dead way then improvisation crept in and she played it again in a really lively way. At the end, she came back again to it in a lively manner. Next she played a Bach Minuet in G and I made encouraging and reassuring comments. The second half was full of mistakes but she sang and kept going. Then I asked her to play just the bass and I took the treble on the violin and she kept going in spite of mistakes. I suggested that she write 4 bars in G with only steps of 1/2 or whole tones. I can't remember why I said this; in fact, although she agreed to try, she never did.

9/6/86. She had played with the cellist but couldn't hear her, and her piano lessons had gone badly. I said that her teacher sounded as if he played totally into her self-punishing side.

I asked her to play, and when she faltered, to start talking about what she felt. She did this, mostly stopping between bars and she said, "It was such a mess." I answered, "You're giving me a mess, a constipated mess. How does sensation rate in your four Jungian functions?" She wept. She felt that she wanted it to be a sensation of caressing the instrument and a kind of special relationship with the composer - a kind of love-making. I commented, "No one must know of this pleasure and instead you produce a mess to hide it." We discussed the possibility of her getting a music therapist as teacher and I gave her a local colleague's address. I felt that she not only wanted to learn to play the piano, but had the need to explore her feelings about learning and expressing her emotions musically. I asked her to be "The Teacher I'd Like." In talking she was kind and directive, the piano playing was wild, she gave wide boundaries as teacher.

7/7/86. She had been for a lakeside holiday. She was to start the next week with a new teacher she had found (not a music therapist). She had played the piano at home with her windows wide open. We improvised on "What I Want to Give My New Teacher." There was multi-instrumental playfulness, yearning, destructiveness and firm assertiveness in her music. We talked about the destructive part and she told me that when she was a pathologist she never completed her research so as to be able to write a paper on it. She said it was laziness. I told her I did not believe in laziness, it is a cosmetically defensive word which provides an excuse for avoiding further exploration of hidden aggression and resistances.

We played about "Completion." She thought of having to relinquish something and finished with a bang on the drum "finishing it off!" We decided to have three more sessions then stop, but I said it was only enough if she continued to play with and to people at home. I said that it was possible that she had feelings about allowing a music therapist to carry out some successful therapy when so much psychotherapy had failed to touch the problem. She agreed.

14/7/86. She had started with her new teacher who was affirmative. She had made lots of mistakes in her Open University theory paper and only managed 47 instead of 80 marks. I felt she needed this area of allowable non-success in her life as previously it had been all success. In this work, unlike in music therapy and piano teaching, she was not getting any help. I thought it could be a sign of strength for her to allow this. We played "Mess" and both made a musical mess.

Then we did "Making Mistakes," she made little tappings on the instruments and sang "I don't know what to do," played melodica clusters and drum, sang "Help," and finished with melodica clusters. Last we improvised "Successful/Unsuccessful," her Successful was not very definite on the xylophone then with single and double notes on the melodica sailing above my "Unsuccessful." Her "Unsuccessful" was chaotic with busy drum, cymbal and xylophone glissandi.

21/7/86. She felt she had let people down: calling the A.A. and then extricating her car, something about a porter and then letting me down because she hadn't played to anyone. However, she had had a good piano lesson focusing on special difficulties and enjoying his jokes. We played "Letting Down/Being Let Down," she felt depressed and helpless in both roles. Her "Letting Down" was rather vague and faint and my "Being Let Down" very angry. My "Letting Down" was quite manic and her "Being Let Down" was slightly more fierce but finishing off with a tremulous melodica tune. Next we played "I Can't." She sang softly with gentle xylophone glissandi then became her angry, destructive super-ego on the double naqqaras, spoiling it.

28/7/86. She told me with some satisfaction that she had practised in the presence of a house guest who was reading, and that

she had had her second piano lesson which had included transposition
and sight-reading. She had decided to learn the recorder again, and
hoped to play with others when her playing improved. Because she
had a definite task to work at I suggested that we should have a follow-
up session on 6/10 and she agreed. She improvised on "Playing As I
Would Like to Play" (on the piano). There were bass chords, plonk,
plonk of free clusters all over the piano. I felt that she was now
"Master of Chaos" and could form it. We improvised imagining there
was "No Music in the World and Then Music Comes." The thought
made her tearful. Her playing and vocalisation was gentle, then
happy, free sounds with bell and cymbal, finishing with drum and
song. She asked me what I felt about the title. I said I felt it was like
not being able to lift up one's heart in the religious sense. She felt it
was important to be playing with people. I said that an audience was
a great resonating chamber like a violin's belly. We finished off with
a black note duet. She felt she did not know the notes well enough to
play freely, but if we could play together often enough, she could. As
we lived in different towns this was difficult but our improvisation
sounded better than it had seemed to her when we played it back.

6/10/86. Follow-up session. She had been playing duets with
her teacher who she experienced as being much better than her former
one. She had played to two new people, though she had to force
herself to do so, and she had played with a recorder-playing elementary pianist. She remembered that her father had had a pupil who he
said would never be able to play Chopin. At once Renata felt she
could never play Chopin. I said she felt she could never be better than
anyone else, Anna or the pupil. She agreed. She told me that her new
teacher chose the Chopin "Raindrops" prelude for her to play and she
felt that after all she could play it. We talked about pentatonic duets
as a prelude to duet playing and we played one with me doing a formal
bass, then one free, then free with her in the bass, and the last, atonal
with a little poaching on each other's territories and much laughter
afterwards. Lastly, we improvised on "Chopin." She played the
instruments. Her playing was amazing because there was a plaintive
melodica tune finding its way into being and then a fierce drum and
cymbal voice and the occasional xylophone. Towards the end there
was the multi-instrumental playing we heard in her "Father" improvisa-

tion earlier. She felt angry at not being able technically to express what she wanted to. She still wasn't sure she could play Chopin. At the end she said that if she got stuck, or if there was something else she couldn't express otherwise, she would come back. Ten months later she invited me to speak at her local Psychotherapy Society, where I showed my video "Music and the Shadow" (see the essay on the same title), and led a discussion which they said they found very stimulating. So it seems as if we are still happily poaching in one another's territories.

I asked the client if she would like to read the case study and write some comments for publication with the paper. Here are her comments on the therapy:

"I cannot recall the work very well but the overall memory is that it was good. I had a sort of childlike delight in being in charge, as it were, in the way that I could influence the mood, rhythm or loudness of the music. I also loved making music with someone. Memorable moments were when I discovered that I could sing and that, to me, my voice sounded clear and an important and integral part of the ensemble of percussion and piano. In two sessions, M.P. talked to me, or rather about me (or so I remember) while I played some easy pieces badly from music which I had brought with me. In one session she denigrated me and that felt deeply familiar, particularly when she said, 'She is so stupid that she doesn't even know what key she is in.' Being called a cow did not bother me, but it was too unlikely. When she praised me, that felt good momentarily but I was not convinced. Maybe it is difficult to praise me."

"An important decision I made during the therapy and I think because of it, was to sack my piano teacher and to find a new one. It dawned on me that I did not <u>have</u> to adapt to something that was so constricting, (and I am sure that I was right in my assessment of the situation)."

"I still have some difficulty in playing in public and I have not practised doing so enough. I have played chamber music with myself on the recorder---no problem---but not with me at the piano--- not yet!"

Stop Press: Yes, she had done this recently, tentatively but with satisfaction.

My summary of our work is as follows: Altogether Renata and

I had 15 analytical music therapy sessions. Many hours of psychotherapy previously had failed to address the problem of playing the piano when anyone was listening. The sessions gradually uncovered Renata's association of music with her intimate phantasy relationship with her father, but because this knowledge was not enough without repeated reality-testing in the present, the sessions continued until her playing and improvising became freer and more enjoyable and she was able to experience elementary chamber music playing to and with friends at which time she felt that the therapy "moved something."

Essay Twenty-Five

Analytical Music Therapy
With Recidivists

Music therapy was started with the recidivists at Camberwell
Day Training Centre (DTC) in March, 1974. The centre was one of
four such alternatives to prison to be initiated in the United Kingdom.
At that time the clients were from 19-45 years of age with IQs from 75
up to the 130s or more. Their offences were mainly theft with some
assault, embezzlement, homosexual soliciting, taking drugs and a few
sexual offences. Previous prison admittance varied from none to
twelve times. The sixty weekdays at the Centre, from nine to five, had
been an alternative to as long as a four year prison sentence. Twelve
years later, writing in Probation Journal (1986) Peter Mark, reported
that in a nine-month follow-up study of one centre, 70% of the men
who attended had not re-offended. Music therapist Sarah Hoskyns,
writing in Psychology of Music (1988) also reported that increased
numbers were released before serving their full sentence.

Each of the three groups of eight men, with their two probation
officers, had one 90-minute music therapy session per week led by
Peter Wright (piano) and myself (violin) as co-therapists, with Marjorie
Wardle (piano) acting as our deputy. Other activities at the Centre
were Art Therapy, Drama, Wrought-Iron Work, Do-It-Yourself, Car
Maintenance, Pottery, Art Development (a kind of pop sculpture)
Playspace (games for adults), Video and Role-play, Gardening,
Gymnastics, small group sessions with the Probation Officers, and
observation outings to places of interest such as museums and
archaeological digs and theatres. There was an opportunity for all the
part-time and full-time staff to get together at a monthly meeting.

We saw the place of music therapy in this therapeutic battery
as being what could be called the soul of the centre. Music is an art
which exercises every part of a person: physical, emotional, mental
and spiritual. Over and above this it takes place dynamically through
the medium of time. This means that it allows for the change of one
emotion into another along with the relaxation which follows tension-
release through this preverbal sound expression. In this it is a unique
therapeutic medium adaptable to the widest range of IQs.

The main functions of our work in the Day Training Centre were to help the clients: 1) to use their "inner space" dynamically as a rehearsal ground for imagined acts and their possible consequences (based on work done with Dr. W. Bion, and more recently Dr. Hyatt Williams at the Tavistock Adolescent Unit); 2) to circumvent blocked verbal expression via release of tension in sound expression producing a more fruitful liason between the unconscious and conscious; 3) to develop a greater degree of group awareness and at least sometimes to experience at first hand a miniature society working in musical and social harmony; 4) to experience socially-acceptable catharsis; 5) to develop awareness of themselves, of their relationships to others and their place in the group as a whole, ever-developing social organism; 6) to learn to bridge the gap between subverbal (body tensions) and verbal expression; 7) to have the experience of taking in noble music under relaxed conditions and to accompany it with their accepted music; and 8) to increase the capacity for reflective thought.

Music therapy took place in a medium-sized upstairs room containing a long table, some chairs, a piano, a cupboard for the instruments and some giant cushions. The instruments we originally bought were a large 3-legged tom-tom, bongos, tambourines, a 16" tambour, a cymbal on a stand, Chinese blocks, a triangle and maraccas and Indian cymbals; but we quickly identified a need to express more tender feelings and so we added a chromatic xylophone, metallaphone, small glockenspiel and an alto melodica of the piano-key variety.

Perhaps the easiest way of describing how we went about trying to exercise the various functions of music therapy is briefly to describe a session---not a typical session, as such a thing did not yet exist---just one particular session.

It is Friday afternoon, a difficult time as the men go down to the Post Office in the lunch hour for their giros and tend to stay down in the pub drinking up the money. This time four men (whom I shall call A, B, C, and D) come back, three stay drinking and one is seeing his solicitor. I sit on the floor with the door open playing the bongos for my own enjoyment. A comes in, grins all over his face, takes the xylophone and joins in. Peter, the two probation officers Brenda and Tad, B and C (who is Carribean black) come in, sit down on the floor and begin to improvise with us on instruments of their choice. C does not play; he looks moody. Tad has previously told me that C has had his best suede coat stolen. We stop. Peter suggests that I play Sibelius' Valse Triste with him and that the others see if they can think of a story while listening. They join in on percussion instruments. I point out that this music is sometimes very soft and suddenly very slow and they will have to be quite sensitive to follow us, which indeed they are and do. A thinks it is some kind of special dance with people getting together and then a tragic end. B thinks that it sounds like someone running away with something and then being caught. C looks surly and doesn't comment. I read the story of the music amid attentive silence. It is clear that C now wants to express something. He mutters something about rats. I suggest that people can sometimes be like rats. "King rats!" he replies and then it bursts out: "Someone took me coat!" With my facilitation he pours out his rage over the theft. "I burn! I burn inside! If I find your coat downstairs I will take it and stamp it in the mud!" I hope I will enable him to fantasise about this (function 1) rather than to hang on to it inside and then act it out in reality. Just then D comes in rather drunk. B tries to reason with C, but C turns on him wild with fury in his pain. When C pauses I say that we are sorry about his best coat, we cannot return it but we do want to help him with his feelings. Peter suggests that we all play "Anger at Things Lost or Stolen."

D sits at the tom-tom and beats all hell out of it. C, who is not playing, gazes at him with an expression of sheer delight, possibly at the freedom of so much fury letting rip in sound. When it is over we share our thoughts about it. C is evasive "I am all right", he says. B was overwhelmed by the drum's sound and gave up his own. A was angry. Behind the anger of loss, Peter says, is a great hurt. C had said he would have given his coat to a man without one if he had asked him for it. He had two other coats. Using the pentatonic scale on the black notes, we all play a long, quiet and very tender piece. I play the violin, muted. C lies relaxed with his head on his giant cushion almost like a babe asleep on the breast. I made a mistake in putting the glockenspiel on the drum for D to play. He is hurt as he regards it as a feminine instrument and refuses to play. When it is over D bursts out that it was like a love song not like hurt. A thinks it was soothing and peaceful. B liked it. Brenda and Tad joined in the playing and responses but I am missing them out for brevity. As we relax on the floor Peter finishes off the session by playing us some Schubert. Deep issues often arise in these sessions and it is then possible for the probation officers to take them further in their thrice-weekly small groups.

The Day Training Centre was part of a three year government experiment; the fact that it is still continuing sixteen years after the end of this period points to an encouraging assessment. It is too early to speak about definitive results as yet but we saw some remarkable developments among the individual men. The rebel leader, who always played the drum fortissimo, became content to take a back seat, achieving a measure of self-containment. The big demolition worker, always arguing and attacking authority, discovered that he could pour out his sadness and the emotional resonances caused by his probation officer going on holiday, into the melodica and make marvellous music. The Caribbean black lad who chose to play a beautfully sensitive melodic "Goodbye" on the metallaphone, found music an easier medium than words for this purpose. Besides these individual changes there are some wonderful musical memories of group improvisations that came alive and came together binding us into a strange whole, breaking down all the barriers of our different roles or reasons for being together.

When I started this work I was frankly apprehensive, not knowing what to expect from the men. Somehow I seemed to imagine that recidivists would be almost like creatures from another planet. But, as with almost everyone else, when you really get to know them you cannot help respecting their essential selves. In fact the "them" disappears as we become "us" with all our different facets and intricate individual patterns of strength and weakness.

However, there are clear musical differences between the playing of these clients at the centre and the psychiatric patients with whom I otherwise work. Most patients are much more free with their imagination and have less difficulty in connecting the inner and outer worlds. Their defences are more subtle and they tend to have better rhythm. I have yet to find a client at the centre with a reliable, generous, springy rhythm; instead you get a dead banging that is very hard to play with and extremely unsettling. On the whole the men have more of a "Full Steam Ahead/Off" polarity in the expression of their drives. It is hard for them to steer a middle course. Nevertheless they produced some delightful sound expressions as they developed this middle area.

The pressure on the music therapists in this work is considerable. We had to be able to contain a great deal of very strong emotion and ride the periods of testing and the power struggles which took place largely in the chaotic element of unstructured sound. At the same time the men's sensitivity and feeling for beauty and the things that make life worthwhile needed also to be allowed to develop. The therapists had to work, too, against the tendency of the clients to avoid thinking in the here-and-now of the session and seeing how present behaviour can be indicative of both past and future trends. Through the clients playing and discussing their feelings, thoughts and inner experiences and being listened to with the therapist's facilitation, each man should, hopefully, by the end of his stay, feel that he had found an accepted and acceptable place in this prototypic group.

We saw our responsibilities as trying to enable enough good experiences to develop in the group to carry the men through their more painful emotional discoveries. We also endeavoured to support those men who went through moments of deep distress, to avoid destructive scapegoating among the men, and to be responsive to their creative leads where possible. In addition, our general aim was, in the words of Dr. D. W. Winnicott, "staying alive, staying awake, and staying well" as far as we could.

The next part of this chapter is based on a second paper, entitled "Music, Freud and Recidivism" which was published in the Journal of the British Society for Music Therapy (1977, 8 [3], 10-13). It also came out in New Society.

In the twenty-three volumes of Freud's complete works he only touches on the subject of criminals 16 times, as against his 672 references to repression and 1,036 to sexual matters. Nevertheless it seemed worthwhile to give some thought to the practical application of one of his theories with reference to the music therapy which Peter Wright and I carried out with recidivists. Therefore I propose to paraphrase one of Freud's theories on criminality, I will then endeavour to show what evidence we saw of this in our therapy, to explain how this worked out in musical improvisation, how the expression of various parts of the personality can be split between the expression in music and words, and finally attempt to formulate the guidelines underlying our contribution to the healing process.

Our music therapy sessions were preceded by a private progress report by the group's two probation officers, and they started and finished with Peter Wright and I playing short pieces of classical music to the men. During the rest of the session we all improvised our own group music on tuned and untuned percussion and simple wind instruments, seated on the floor in the Eastern manner. Sometimes our music was pure sound expression, playing with rhythm and textures, but often it was the accompaniment to an inner exploration on a mutually agreed subject such as "The Job I Want," "A Load of Shit," or "My earliest Memory." And this brings us back to Freud.

In "Dostoevsky and Parricide" (Volume 21 of the Complete Works, p. 177-194), Freud wrote that a considerable portion of criminals actually want to be punished as this saves them from punishing themselves in some way via their own super-egos. Previously he had written a short paper entitled "Criminals from a sense of guilt" (Volume 14 of the Complete Works, p. 332-336) in which he described a person who was suffering from an oppressive feeling of guilt, the origin of which was unknown to him. After he had committed some crime this uncomfortable feeling abated somewhat as it was now at least connected to something known to him. How, in our music therapy, were we made aware of this sense of guilt which indeed with recidivists persists beyond the one crime and leads on to the next and the next? In four main ways, which however, only applied to about fifty percent of the offenders who we saw. The sense of guilt: A) forbids any inner rehearsal of offences; B) brings with it a very poor self-image; C) forbids the imagination of receiving good things; and D) causes the men violently to resist using their own creativity.

Our method of working was to let an imagination exercise be accompanied by musical expression of the feelings evoked. We taped the music and after we had talked about our inner experiences we listened to the group musical expression and discussed that.

The following are the musical and verbal expressions

accompanying exercises revealing these four ways that show the men's guilt feelings.

In an exercise showing "A" (no inner rehearsal of offences), the men were to imagine travelling a long way to a friend's house on a cold, wet night, seeing lights on, knocking and ringing and getting no reply and then reacting violently. There was tremendous power and pace in their music which seemed to be a group expression. However, half of the group were quite unable to imagine anything at all, among them two of the most violent men. Of the others, two fantasised blowing up the house (one imagined being arrested), and another smashed all the windows saying that his friend was in there "screwing." When I went to play back the tape, the men were horrified to think that this wild music had been recorded. As a matter of fact I had pressed the wrong button and it had not been recorded.

In an exercise showing "B" (poor self-image), the men were asked to imagine meeting themselves for the first time, as a stranger might. Their musical expression was an excited drumming so that the subsequent depressive description of the unpleasant people that they considered themselves to be, came as quite a surprise. Only one man was very defended against such feelings and thought himself splendid in every way. Whether his music was depressive I did not notice.

In an exercise showing "C" (no imagination of receiving good things), they picked cards on the reverse sides of which were written sums from £1 up to £100,000,000 which they were to imagine that they had won. There was thrumming excitement again in the noisy music which did not match their words at all. Half could not imagine anything and the others were expressing contempt for any sum under £10,000. This sum was imagined to have limitless purchasing power. Their fear of envy permitted all but one to desire only a "little house" if they had won the top prize.

In contrast with this was our experience with the remains of a group whose other more disturbed members had dropped out or been taken into custody. Their music gently bubbled along with an eager drumming and one single cymbal clash. One man fantasised giving his £100 to his children (he was divorced); another put his £10 on a horse (the drumming), won £100 (the cymbal) with which he bought carpets and curtains for his "pad;" the third stretched his £10,000 to include a house, car, gardening business and rich presents to the Centre and his probation officer. Here creativity had begun to creep in.

As for "D" (resisting creativity), there were protracted arguments about the usefulness of the therapy. When they did consent to play, about half the men at first had only the aim of destroying the whole session by sheer volume of sound, two or three competing to be the leaders. The reaction-formation to this was taking the tiny Indian cymbals, the handbells or a triangle so that they could not damage anyone with their impulses.

By now it may seem that half of the men were just unable to fantasise while they played. But this was not the case. No one failed to produce an "Earliest Memory" or was unable to imagine a job that he wanted to do. This seemed to be contradictory at first but it was only that in certain areas, for example crime, there was an inability to use their imagination.

It may sound as if their music was just noisy. But neither was this the case. Although a lot of their music was noisy, it was not always so. These improvisations contrasted, for example, with one starting with listening in silence to the sounds coming from the wind in the branches outside the window. Here delicate textures of sound and rhythmic interplay developed and then faded into careful listening. In an improvisation on "Silence and Sound," each man held back until he felt there was space for his expression and the lacy texture of the musical fabric was a joy to hear.

In these two last improvisations the men seemed to be functioning in an integrated way, whereas in the previous four examples their splits were acted out between the music and the words. I will explain this:

In "A" the music expressed the aggressive impulse but in the words of half the men, the consciousness of the impulse was lacking.

In "B" the words represented their depression about themselves, and the music the manic defence that habitually covered this depression up with apparently light-hearted behaviour and refusal to take anything seriously.

In "C" as in "A," the music represented the impulse, here greedy, but the words expressed their defences, the denial of this impulse, the contempt for the prizes, the fear of envy and the suppression of all greed but the modest wish for a little house.

In "D" they themselves were playing the part of their punitive super-egos, from which they regularly dissociated when committing their offences by projecting them on to policemen and other authority figures. They projected on to their therapists that part of themselves which might be usefully and fruitfully creative if only they could allow it to be. The main aim of the therapists in this case was to prove that this creative part could survive the super-ego attacks and later to reverse the roles but offer the men a more tolerable version of a super-ego for introjection.

It is exceedingly difficult to help recidivists of this kind to help themselves, but we believed that this work could, and sometimes did, contribute towards a lessening of their oppressive feeling of guilt in the following ways. It helped them: to integrate by accepting, because we accepted via the music and words, all their feelings instead of denying some and acting them out in crime; to trust in their own creativity which, though musical, could carry over into other spheres of life; to interact spontaneously and sensitively in a musico-social setting; to have a sense of personal value and thus obtain some hope of feeling worthy of good experiences; and to increase their ability to use their "inner space" to rehearse criminal (and other) actions (as law-abiding people do) so that they could relieve their feelings enough to be able to think of the possible consequences and decide on alternate actions.

I will close with a final paraphrase of Freud's "The Ego and the Id" (Volume 19 of the Complete Works, p. 19-27). He wrote that especially in young criminals one could detect a strong sense of guilt which had preceded their crime and was therefore not its consequence but its motive. It was for the benefit of such young people that we particularly directed our efforts towards the practical application of this theory.

The views put forward in this chapter were not necessarily those held by the other staff at the Day Training Centre, either then or now.

Essay Twenty-Six

Preliminary Music

I started Preliminary Music with the thought of giving intelligent "normal" children aged about four to six years the opportunity to explore sounds and rhythms on my forty different fairly primitive musical instruments before starting their formal instrumental instruction. Sessions are in half-hour periods once weekly. My instruments are quite simple and are mostly of the kind that have been used in religious and healing ceremonies all over the world for thousands of years.

My deepest thought was that music is a language---a language of the emotions. From my own experience I had discovered that languages taught in the classroom in my childhood in meaningless lists of verb-conjugations to be learnt by rote with a perfect accent, do not stick in the mind as something that one can use. Whereas languages learnt in countries where even an approximation of their regional sounds produces meaningful results in the way of exchanges of goods, information or pleasant greetings, stick in the mind as useful tools free from inhibiting memories of boredom or embarrassment.

Then why not let children find their own meaningful music, expressing their emotions through experimental self-created sounds and rhythms? Let them go back through a philogenic experience discovering that "This sound is my own, it is what I mean or feel at this moment in time and I am with someone who understands it." The idea was born when I started letting little violin pupils have a space for free-play on my instruments as a treat or carrot at the end of their lessons. The results were delightful and an obedient apathetic little pupil could sometimes suddenly turn into a master of dynamic and meaningful creativity. The key that opened this amazing door seemed to be creative play.

I visualised the attraction for the fee-paying parent as a course of twelve weekly sessions with a written assessment of the child's musical aptitude and preference of instrumental type at the end of this period. However, things worked out very differently. I had not reckoned with the deep and far-reaching power of self-creativity through playing. Nor had I reckoned with the thoroughgoing work done by Ben-Tovim and Boyd (1985) regarding the mental and physical requirements for professional success on a given instrument being weighed up with the emotional and symbolic satisfaction that a self-chosen instrument could give to a young child who was probably going to be a satisfied amateur musician.

The children and their mothers came to me via a small advertisement in the local music shop. On my headed notepaper it offered Violin Tuition, beginners to advanced, Music Therapy for emotional problems, and Preliminary music for children from 4 to 6 years of age. I did not have any prior interview with the parents when I began this work and so did not in every case know that some of the children had been quite seriously school phobic at the start of our work, beginning every schoolday with tears. However, I have subsequently instigated a short questionnaire to be filled in initially by the parent, with the child in the room either fiddling about with the instruments or sitting forlornly on the floor looking at them. The reaction to this situation, plus the information in the questionnaire, told me something about the parent-child relationship. It is followed by a short assessment session with the child, to see if we can get on with each other. A questionnaire sent to the mothers at the end of these sessions told me that, in fact, the mothers had sent their children to me because of my music therapy qualification in the advertisement. However, as in this country the greatest share of music therapy goes to mentally-handicapped children, many parents do not like it to be known that their brilliant child is going to "therapy." But the title Preliminary Music was acceptable.

As regards the therapeutic aspect of play, which in my opinion is equally valid for all ages, I will quote two excerpts from Dr. D. W. Winnicott's book, Playing and Reality: "It is in playing and only in playing that the individual or adult is able to be creative and to use the whole personality, and it is only in being creative that the individual discovers the self" (p. 63). And later: "We find either that individuals live creatively and feel that life is worth living or else that they cannot live creatively and are doubtful about the value of living" (p. 83). Opposed to this creative living he saw a life of compliance and adaptation. The unexpected results of Preliminary Music certainly rendered me adaptive but the outcome was creative for the children, their parents and ultimately for me, because it made me think.

In the afternoon session, I had no particular aims for the child but would try and help him to pursue his own aims and interests in an atmosphere of play. It is important to realise that play can also be deep seriousness with the "shoulds" and "oughts" taken out. Unlike some therapists I answered every question the child asked, as simply and as honestly as I could. I paid close attention to him in his activity and the thought and emotion inherent in it, for a concentrated half hour. It was exhausting, especially in the beginning when children's concentration spans were so short and they jumped rapidly from one sphere of interest to another. Also I really do believe that timewise a small child's half hour is much longer than the half hour of a person fifty or sixty years older.

I did not regard my role as being a therapist in the usual sense of the word but did see our sessions as being therapeutic. My role was akin to being the Joker in a pack of cards. I was alternately observer, listener, audience, accompanist, cassette recorder operator, security officer for persons and property, teacher, pupil, playmate, the mirrorer of emotions and the introducer of the odd complementary or compensatory idea. Up to a point I could be manipulated and used in any way the child wanted. Beyond that point boundaries were reliably firm. Keeping the work within the half hour was one boundary and the other was the rule that the child should not damage the instruments, him/herself or me.

The surprising result of the sessions with the three first intelligent "normal" children who I will later describe, was that they used these half hours to work out their own pressing problems, which in two cases were preventing their smooth development and educational progress. The first child used the time to adapt to her feelings about her mother's pregnancy by her stepfather and the forthcoming arrival of her first sibling. The second used the time to let both of us know that she had an artistic and creative self and that she felt miserable in her uncomfortable environment. This concluded with the alteration of these circumstances without any direct interference from me. The third child used the time to make the transition from being an anxious only son of a worried career-driven mother, to being a confident member of his male peer group, feeling that it was at last safe to allow himself to be taught a few basic skills, and happy now to have his mother at home.

By their twelfth sessions I could see that important processes had started and it would be criminal just to tell the parents that we would break off the work there. Besides which, the children were so keen to come somewhere where they felt they were free to be themselves; and the mothers so glad to see their children happier, that it would have been difficult for the parents to stop the work at that point.

Although the subsequent questionnaire showed that some parents would have liked an initial explanatory interview, I felt at the time that there can be an advantage in leaving things a bit vague inside and outside at times, and gave none.

I have thought hard about what enabled these externally and internally creative and healing processes to happen. I put it down to three factors: the teleological (goal-seeking) child with his/her goal of wholeness; the presence of objects to play with; and the close personal attention of an adult who is willing to believe that the child's activities have meaning and value even if she does not always know exactly what the meaning is at any given moment.

The years around four to six have special value in this connection. According to Erich Neumann (1973), the first year is a post-uterine embryonic phase. For the next two years the child is emotionally and mentally very much contained by the mothering person. If she is cooking then he wants to cook, if she is crying then he will cry too. Her values are his credo, her moods his weather. Then, jumping to the age of seven, he is now largely contained by the peer group. He must look like them, talk like them, play like them and live like them. But in the years between, from roughly four to six, we have the Golden Years, a most valuable remedial and preventive period when the child can be in a free and flexible state. At this time he is able to play creatively through the less seriously traumatising difficulties of his life which, however, could well produce a warped adaptation to life, taking years to remedy therapeutically at a much later date. It is in this Golden period that a child can show startling originality in thought and deed. If these clues are recognised and fostered they can be a vital pointer to the successful future navigation of his life's journey.

Sometimes a parent is so concerned about how she thinks the child ought to be that she fails to pick up these cues and even dampens the vital sparks that a teacher or near relative may be able to see. For example, the mother of the boy in the third case study complained that her son learned nothing in school but only daydreamed. In my flat he showed himself voraciously hungry for knowledge: "What is that? How does it work? May I see it? Touch it?" He wanted to explore everything. His mother would say "Not so many questions! His curiosity is terrible," her anxiety about the development of good manners scotomising the very springs of learning at source. The end of term reports on our progress were able to make some useful links for the parents who confirmed this in the questionnaire. However, perhaps I should have been more direct in putting my ideas to some of the parents. But I thought the danger of making the mothers distrust their own good feeling of parenthood (so easily undermined in these days of experts) and act at secondhand from outside advice, would be the greater danger and so said nothing. Besides, being a parent and grandparent oneself produces a certain amount of healthy humility.

Preliminary Music only caters for children on a one-to-one basis because the therapist must be so carefully attuned to the child's feelings and ideas, often expressed through movement as much as through speech or musical activity. I, personally, have avoided seeing two children from the same family to avoid rivalry and jealousy, of which they usually have enough already.

Katy

Katy was just five years old when she came to Preliminary Music. She was a happy child with plump, red cheeks and thick sandy-coloured hair. Her parents were divorced, father lived abroad and mother had recently re-married. Altogether Katy had 33 sessions over 13 months. In her 1st session she played with excellent rhythm, inventing a song about her relative falling off a donkey called Jose. In sessions 2 and 3, her improvisations and songs became a bit longer. In 4, I showed her the cards with note values and she played these correctly on the violin to her mother. I do not usually allow the mothers in, but Katy pleaded most earnestly for her mother to come in, so I allowed her in at half time. Katy explored more of the forty instruments as we progressed. In session 9, she came in hopping like a frog and I accompanied her with hopping music. She made mysterious footstep sounds with the wire brush on the drum and a story about a monster, perhaps her greedy-baby self.

In session 11, playing the chordal dulcimer, she discovered, with interest and delight, that she could play louder with her nail and could stop the vibration by touching the string. In our dyadic first half of the session I mirrored her pleasure at her discovery, so she showed her mother Jane this when we were the trio in the second half, clearly hoping for the same response. However, sad to say, Jane did not react at all to the excitement of the discovery. In fact throughout the session Jane looked a bit uncomfortable at Katy's behaviour, probably not knowing what she should be doing, and feeling a bit guilty and responsible in case she was not doing the right thing. Perhaps I should have made some explanation on the phone afterwards, but I felt at the time like leaving things to develop in a natural way and not to try to make anything happen willfully. I felt instinctively that Katy knew the way forward if she was given a chance, and the less I interfered the better. However, I did not feel that my belief was yet backed up by the kind of rational explanations that might convince her mother who was paying for this treatment. So I kept quiet.

In session 13, Katy brought her doll Rosie for the first time. I thought this significant, and in fact Jane must have been planning her new baby at that time. In sessions 14 and 15, Katy became a hopping frog and squirming snake on the Turkish prayer rug while I accompanied her on the piano. Could she be in touch with the developing child in her mother's womb, I wondered?

After their next holiday abroad her behaviour to her mother changed. She was the mature little musician with me; and a very clinging baby when Jane came in. After session 18, I wrote in my diary, "I wonder if Jane is pregnant." Katy had been hopping like a frog and then sat on Jane's lap with her doll saying solemnly, "It wasn't a frog." She seemed aware, at a deep level, of the new life which took up some of her mother's attention. From session 19, she started to play known tunes by ear on the piano and melodica. She showed unusually powerful and lengthy concentration and determination. It was almost as if she were thinking "If there is going to be a new arrival in this family, he or she is going to find someone here to be reckoned with."

In session 23, she sat on her mother's lap pretending to be a suckling baby. By this time Jane seemed to get some inkling of what was going on; and though looking a bit embarrassed, taking her cue from me, allowed Katy to express these thoughts in action with gentle understanding, either conscious or unconscious. Katy dismembered the xylophone to find the lost beater's head which had flown off. What mother had inside her could not be investigated so easily. In a song she sung "my little brother comes to tea." Her music became more ambitious. I was very glad when in one session her mother was with us and Katy did some really amazingly beautiful xylophone improvisations with my piano accompaniment. I did not have the cassette recorder going at the right moment, and recording all the sessions would have been too expensive for me at that time, so it remains only in our memories.

By session 28, Jane's belly was huge and Katy did a beautiful dance with her mother's scarf. She began to show a feeling of loving responsibility for her mother, and in session 29, Katy involved all three of us in a chime bar improvisation for the first time. We made some cassette recordings and she became very squeaky and excited. On one tape I played for her maracca dance and when the bell went she sang a song she wanted me to hear, very fast to get it all in. (I use a timer for children's sessions because of the intense involvement and the difference in the time-feeling in the different ages).

Session 30 was important for Katy. She solemnly and deliberately took one instrument after another over to Jane and arranged them around herself until she was playing twelve instruments at once. Jane seemed somehow embarrassed and uneasy about this but I understood Katy as convincing herself, in a magical way, that if she could play 12 instruments at once then her mother could easily care for her, her stepfather and the new baby or babies that her mother contained.

During the last three sessions, Katy showed tender maternal (or perhaps paternal) concern for her mother, involving her lovingly in our music, and organising our trio on the chime bars as a farewell piece. Jane, for her part, was losing her social persona and merging into a more gentle and vulnerable state of mind. As Katy had been born after only half an hour's labour, Jane dared not risk the car journey to my flat four weeks from the expected birthday, so we parted. Georgina was born four weeks later and Jane wrote that Katy had shown no disturbance or resentment at the arrival of her half-sister. Katy started piano lessons at the beginning of the next term and at the follow-up five years later she had taken her Grade 5 on the piano and 4 on the cello. And she had another little half-sister.

Katy had had a good start experiencing the value of music as a conveyor of deep personal meaning and expression, and she had used it to help herself through a difficult adjustment and transition from being "only child" in one family to being the big sister in another.

Zoe

Zoe was a blue-eyed, pink-cheeked little girl with long golden ringlets and the appearance of a disgruntled doll. Sometimes she came to her session with her Nanny, sometimes with her continental grandmother, sometimes with a family friend, once with her separated father, occasionallly with her working mother, and sometimes in a huge limousine whose chauffeur waited for her in the car outside my basement flat reminding me of my own childhood.

At the start of our work she was five years old and I found out later that she had been crying every day when it was time for her to go to her French-language school. The period of work discussed incorporated 33 sessions over 16 months. At the first session at 4 PM, she refused to enter the flat and sat down on the stone steps leading down to my front door. Her mother came in and talked to me for ten minutes. After that time I suggested that she tell Zoe that we would sit there until 4:30 PM when she and her mother would go home but if she wanted to come in before that she could. The mother went out and Zoe came in to go to the toilet then sat oustide my workroom in the passage. I began to play the piano in the sad and rather resigned Dorian mode. Zoe came in and offered me a peppermint which I accepted. After that she played on various drums accompanied by me on the piano, and I stopped the session sharp at 4:30 PM when the next child came.

For the next two sessions Zoe explored the instruments and recorded some little French songs in rather a tense, neat fashion. She had learnt them at school. Her concentration span was short but she enjoyed a spell of our copying each other's rhythms on drums. In session 4, she danced beautifully to my piano music and recorded a song with more expression using some instruments. She started to control me saying, "Don't play the piano when I sing, it makes it more difficult." So I didn't! In session 5, after playing the xylophone, melodica and bells, she drew a crenellated castle and asked me not to play the piano meanwhile. So I didn't!

Session 8 was very dramatic. She sat drawing but wanted me to sit motionless at the piano staring at the corner of the room. When I moved and played a note to see what she would do, she came and smacked me and said I was naughty, her little face contorted with rage. I said, "I wonder who did that to you." "My Nanny," she paused, "And my Mummy." After that I was forbidden to move. "It seems like you want me to be dead," I said. Then she came and played on the piano and allowed me to play. She wanted the television on but I said no, we made our own music in her time with me.

Session 9 was the beginning of musical games in which she controlled me but in a more acceptable fashion. We played "Statues" and "Hunt the Bell." In "Statues" she danced round till the music stopped and then froze immobile and I had to guess what she was pretending to be. In "Hunt the Bell" I played the xylophone with my eyes shut while she hid the bell and then I had to find it while she played. In session 10, she clung to her mother in a fury and refused to come in. After a few minutes I said, "She'll be all right now." Her mother left, and Zoe kicked wildly and screamed. I held her gently but firmly. "When you are cross you feel like a little animal. What sort is it?", I asked. She talked about her pets. We had a good session after that, with singing and playing.

In session 11, she played the psaltery carefully and told me about her strict school teacher who gave them written instructions and would not answer questions. (Remember she was just 5). We played the piano and drums together. I found she responded more to minor keys. In session 14, for the last time she sat in the car and refused to come out. I told her I had something new in the room and she came in and chose colours on the new Hygeia colour lamp. The controlling musical games continued but now without any sadism.

In session 15, her hair was straight, the lovely ringlets gone. The Nanny had been sacked. The controlling games continued. In session 17, a new Nanny came. In 18, she told a story of a man taking a girl from her school playground into a taxi and cutting her throat: "It is my little sister and Mummy doesn't know and she will come and find her gone." When her little sister did come to fetch her with the new Nanny I kept her out of our work room and later, when her mother asked for the little one to begin sessions, I said I only take one child from a family for Preliminary Music. Zoe needed someone to be just for her.

The controlling games became more musical and more creative, Zoe became wonderfully sensitive to my loud or soft drumming as she approached or distanced herself from the hidden bell. In session 25, she had an earache and was off school, but had insisted on coming to music. She saw me practising my violin through the window of my basement flat and played on the quarter-sized violin, with me on the piano. In 27, she was very angry and demanding as a teacher who wanted me to copy her music. I had a strong countertransference experience of overwhelming fear and confusion at my inability to do it right, and told her this in simple words as I felt it was her unspoken reaction to her school situation which she could not communicate as forcefully in any other way.

Between sessions 28 and 29, she had her adenoids out and came straight back into the controlling games; but afterwards drew a picture, shouting out the subjects as she drew them so I could improvise to them on the piano. The games continued but one day she demanded different colours from the lamp in operatic singing, beautifully pitched (unlike her French songs) and I had to improvise "colour music." This development continued until the end of our work.

Session 33 was the last one. Her mother showed me the prospectus of a new school which seemed to offer a more gently artistic and progressive approach. Zoe had bashed the cymbal repeatedly singing, "I'm never, ever, ever going to that school again!" It was actually of impeccable reputation but more for the tough than tender-minded. I never mentioned the Nanny and the school to her mother and wondered what had taken place between them to release Zoe from that bondage. I felt that our work had gradually unfrozen the defences of that castle, created by an unhappy situation, revealing a creative and artistic nature and a happier child and mother. Five years later she was still at the new school, happy and much more comfortable in her relationships.

Frank

Frank was 5 years and 10 months old when he came for Preliminary Music. He had over 47 sessions in 18 months. He was very sensitive, pale, fair, intelligent and extremely interested in how the instruments were constructed and how they produced sounds. His concentration span at first was only a few seconds long and his mind was in a whirl. His mother was French, a teacher probably in her late thirties, who constantly warned him against damaging things. His father was a successful business man also from the continent. His mother said that he cried every day when he had to go to school and the teacher said that he dreamed all the time when he was there.

For the first six sessions he explored and played the violin, Chinese blocks, xylophone, raft zither, bells and cymbal. In the second session he dared to play the cymbal very loudly, seeming relieved to cause neither damage nor scolding. In 6, he asked me to work the bull-roarer, an instrument originally shaped like a fish on a string, formerly used in manhood initiation rites for youths. This is an instrument which can cause damage to the player or the environment. Although I would trust giving it to my own children to play with under supervision, I have since taken it out of the workroom armoury. Frank had a tentative try at it but could not make the bull-roaring sound and gave up. His mother asked whether I could now teach him something. I answered, "He needs a playground, he is very much alive and in reality here, not dreaming at all."

In session 7, she said his reading was better and things were clearing up for him. From this time he began to tell me things that had happened at home and we improvised music to them as well as to his invented stories. For example: his friend had tadpoles; a dog bit him; and he lost his mother in the supermarket.

In session 16, his mother again asked if he was ready to learn, she meant be formally taught. I said not yet but we did do some drumming and violin playing to different note values. I asked him if he would like to learn a piece on the piano and he said "No." He said he wanted to play from real music but in fact only wanted to choose some sheet music to put on the stand while he drummed. He started to think creatively about what he wanted to do in his half hour and would collect a battery of instruments round the cassette recorder with concentration and perseverance. Sometimes the time was up before he actually began to play. In session 19, he chose yellow on my new colour lamp and from then on put it on at the beginning of every session.

Before session 23, his mother said that he was much happier at school and his reading had improved. In 25, he wanted to learn a piece on the melodica and I taught him the first phrases of Frere Jacques. After 27, his mother said his maths grades were better.

In 30, he said that he was going to Scouts now and that he wanted to learn the trumpet as his friend played it. I didn't have a trumpet, partly because I was afraid the neighbours might complain, partly because I don't like the sound, and partly because the modern trumpet is not primitive enough for the immediate satisfaction through sound expression that I want for the children in these sessions. At this time his rhythm was generally very poor and he took no delight in it; but he did enjoy our dyadic drum arguments and conversations.

In session 32, his mother said that all his grades were now Bs and Cs where they had been Ds. We had had a real battle to give him the freedom to play, and his ability to choose to reject teaching consciously and in words, seemed to set him free to ask to be taught when he did feel like it. He told me that he had been to Cubs and was frightened at first. He said he always squeaked on the violin and I showed him how to avoid this.

In session 36, he just sat still for several minutes and thought hard about what he wanted to do. He told me that he had been given 19 out of 20 for Biology. At last he could find somewhere where his curiosity about how things were made came in useful. He got out the chime bars and experimented alone very systematically and intelligently in releasing and stopping the sound. In 37, he said he didn't want to go to boarding school as he would miss his Mum. In session 38, he again said that he wanted to learn the trumpet. I explained that I did not know how to play a trumpet and that I still did not have one.

After 40, his mother said that she would arrange for a half hour trumpet lesson at school but still wanted his Preliminary music sessions to continue. In 42, he played the Chinese blocks, we had a conversation on triangles and afterwards he said that his first trumpet lesson had been "OK."

In session 43, he brought his trumpet and we recorded an improvisation. There was a lot of musical fumbling around and finally he triumphantly played a clear high note. By now he was a confident peer-group member, concentrated, decisive and purposeful. He told me anxiously that the teacher had played on his (Frank's) trumpet and he was afraid of germs. We told his mother this after the session and she was shocked because Frank had said that the teacher had used a separate mouthpiece. Frank had been afraid that if he told the truth his mother would stop the lessons. His mother said that she would sort this out with the teacher.

In session 44, he played two string ostinatos on the violin and we played some pleasant duets. I think that by then he could distinguish the way the Preliminary Music session was conducted from the discipline of the trumpet lesson.

By the 47th session, Frank showed curiosity and great pleasure in the process of exploring. To me, this seems to be the raw material for all learning, to the point at school where anatomical curiosity can pass into science and biology, curiosity about our forbears can be satisfied in history, of exploring by geography, of fondling and handling in art, woodwork and music.

For me the moving thing about Preliminary Music is what powerful and preventive effects this one little half hour weekly of undivided attention can facilitate, through attempting to allow the child to find its own personal meaning through its musical play. Perhaps it can be explained also in another quotation from Erich Neumann (1973): "Only an individual embedded in this symbolic reality of play can become a complete human being. One of the main dangers implicit in this modern, occidental-patriarchal culture with its overaccentuation of rational consciousness and its one-sided extraverted adaptation to reality, is that it tends to damage, if not destroy, this pregnant and sustaining symbol world of childhood. "

The crucial thing for the music therapist doing this work, is to have his own inner world of childhood and creativity acting daily as a nourishing force in his life.

Essay Twenty-Seven

Analytical Music Therapy With Children

Given a "good enough" parental couple, and the company of peers by the second half of the second year, most children will work through their difficulties and anxieties in the context of play. This is the play that Winnicott (1971) describes as a self-healing kind. For example, after painful interviews with the doctor (or surgery), a child may subject her teddy bears, pets or younger siblings to lengthy and horrific examinations, while identifying completely with the doctor. Being now in this powerful position she can allay the new victim's fears, and express some of the sadism she felt was directed at her: "It won't hurt once we've got your leg off. Don't wriggle so!"

Often, when she becomes a member of a little group, she can work through her problem by proxy with another child in the role that she would like, and will probably see that she gets, when she has a more dominant position in a subsequent group. As an example of how magical wishes can be used in play I will cite the experiences of two young sisters, Tessa and Nanette, who had a long series of games involving pretending to make a marvelous medicine in discarded household jars in a pigeon house which they called the Stink House. Behind this lengthy game, which took weeks or even months to work through, was at any rate Nanette's wish that she might miraculously heal her mother and avoid the parents' long winter peregrinations to sunny climates in search of health, which left the children in the care of the Nanny whom Nanette hated. The Stink House was so-called because it was unconsciously felt that it was Nanette's own sadistic faecal attacks that had damaged her mother in the first place. The fantasy was possibly shared but it was only Nanette who was later analysed.

Children are acting out their fantasies in this way all the time, working them through in play. It is only when they get trapped in them and cannot develop any further that their learning and behaviour suffers and they need help.

Therefore the analytical music therapist's aim with a child-patient is to restore to her, or introduce to her, the ability to involve herself in the important "work" of self-healing play, together with the freedom to use her natural curiosity and creativity. As Winnicott (1971) wrote, "playing has a place and a time" (p. 47). The analytical music therapy session provides the place and time at first. As far as possible the session resembles a series of games arising, or partly arising, from the child's imagination. I say partly because at first some children's fantasies are so repressed that it may be necessary for the therapist to "get in at the back" and fish one out to be played about. Such repressed fantasies can cause a great deal of guilt and lead the child to act in a punishment-seeking way. They can also be so savage that similar sadism is credited to the mother's body (the infant's first environment), so that this cannot be explored in fantasy and anything that becomes a symbol of this is similarly taboo. Thus the child suffers an inhibition of learning, and withdraws its interest from the outside world. Melanie Klein (1931) wrote: "When, however, the super-ego exerts a too extensive domination over the ego, the latter frequently, in its attempts to maintain control over the id and the internalized objects by repression, shuts itself off from the influences of the outer world and objects there, and thus deprives itself of all sources of stimulus which would form the basis of ego-interests and achievements both those from the id and those from external sources."

If the pair can play their way forward with stories and music, and accommodation to the fantasies of the child, then there may be no need for interpretation at all, but where the child is inextricably trapped in a repeated story it may be possible for the therapist, where he understands what is being expressed, to link this to her reality situation and shape up a sequel. What is needed is that the child should evolve a fruitful interaction between conscious and unconscious. In fact she needs to learn to play. At all events it is essential that any interpretation should not be given in such a way that the child regards it as a criticism of her productions and the creativity is withered away.

There are important differences between working with children and adults. Klein found that in carrying out analysis with children their free play with toys had to take the place of adult verbal free association because of their inability to talk about thoughts and feelings directly. In analytical music therapy with children between two and twelve, the musical story takes the place of the free play with toys. In their sessions, most children need to act and express feelings in this way immediately and not wait until later on in the session like an adult patient who often needs to be warmed up to the point of being able to improvise. The whole action of the therapy seems to be speeded up in the case of a child. One expression succeeds another on their faces much faster than with most adult patients, especially when they are on prescribed drugs.

The duet improvisation has the power to allow the child to enter into his emotions more deeply and purposively and to persevere in his improvisation with increased concentration. It also serves to meet the childish omnipotence as a little thump on the xylophone or blast on the melodica becomes transformed into beautiful (or ugly), powerful and satisfying music by the therapist's skill and empathetic imagination. I think it is at this point that the child's music could be called a transitional phenomenon belonging partly to his own imagination and needs, and partly to the larger reality of the improvisatory duet.

Although I have not, personally, done much long-term work with children, trial sessions with individual children have yielded interesting results. Here are some notes on these sessions, with comments.

Marie was three years old and in the phase of experiencing mother as an uncomfortable rival for father's attention. Marie was attracted to the gong and hit it repeatedly with crows of delight. What this symbolised, shortly became reality when she hit her mother sharply and purposely on the head with the gong stick. Her mother was angry and indignant, and Marie subsequently felt even her symbolic attacks on the gong to be daring and a bit frightening. She had a salutory lesson in the difference between symbol and reality.

Tracey was four, a Singalese child adopted into a British family where there was a six year old daughter. Tracey wanted to play the music of a story about a kitten who died from eating glass and a friendly bird who ate a violin and died. Her playing was very free, she smashed aggressively at the cymbal with a sweep of the arm in between playing on the xylophone with no trace of the pulling back and wincing that Marie (now 6) showed. Instruments were bashed and shaken freely without any worry about what their names might be or what the normal way of using them was. From playing she went into a kind of dance. A "horrible lady" was a xylophone glissando and a "horrible stepmother" walking over the road was expressed by the two beaters clashed together over her head. As I played her very passionate (by countertransference) music, she did a most beautiful, exotic dance with her head turned to one side, her eyes half closed and her little arms up above her shoulders. From being the beady-eyed, rather hunched up little sister, she took on an almost queenly aspect. When she finished, she told me this story and added that a giant mouse fell out of father's bed.

The Jungian analyst to whom I played her music and recounted the story said he thought she had a sexual disturbance. Her mother was, in fact, worried by her continual masturbation and decided to get some help for her.

Marie was now six, a violinist with an acute ear, and a sensible, practical approach to life. Marie had little feeling for the continuity of rhythm. If there was something to be thought out she would stop and set her intelligent little brain to it until she had puzzled it out. Then she would start to play again. After we had improvised our story we played about a bit together. Her fortissimo cymbal clashes were played tensely with a good deal of fear and mirth at the daringness of her explosions. She explored the unusual instruments, wanting first to know their names and then how to play them. She entered into a relationship with the instruments in a rational manner. Marie's story was to be about a wolf who chased a pigeon. "Do you begin first?" she asked, wanting to do it properly. "No, you begin, I'll follow." After some music she stopped and said, "I want the music to go faster and faster." I obliged and as the crescendo reached its height she played a mezzo-forte bang on the drum which she said afterwards was the wolf leaping up into the tree to get the pigeon's egg for his supper. I think that the power of our crescendo was a little frightening for her as she broke off rather suddenly with a shrinking up and a giggle saying she was afraid that we would wake the neighbours if we went on. It was interesting that Marie, who ate almost no tea, should portray herself as a ravening wolf. She was probably already in the latency period by now, managing to sublimate her drives but she nevertheless expressed quite a lot of feeling in her music. She appeared to have some anxiety about using her aggression, no doubt linked to her early fantasies as the one described before when she attacked her mother. Both children loved the sessions and begged to be allowed to stay.

From the practical point of view, it is extremely helpful to have the piano turned at an angle that allows the therapist to see the child, as he may sometimes partly be accompanying a dance which may give a clearer idea of the child's rhythmic sense than her actual playing does.

Annabelle, a child of eight, came in to her first pre-instrumental session with her overly forthright, seemingly insensitive mother. At first the mother, who was out of work, was going to send the child with her au pair but I said I thought Annabelle might feel more at ease at first in a place which her mother had seen. "Annabelle takes these things in her stride," she said; but she nevertheless agreed to come along the first time. It seemed that weakness, sensitivity and anxiety were excluded from the family repertoire of emotions. When she left, and Annabelle had explored the instruments gently, I suggested that Annabelle might make up a story that we could play about with music. In her mother's hard tone she said, "I couldn't do anything like that." I suggested nevertheless that we recorded some music together and maybe a story would come. She started off on the melodica trying to play "Frere Jacques," but improvised freely after the first wrong note; her music started cheerfully in 4/4 with little rhythmic phrases, which I echoed on the piano. Towards the end, the gap between what she could do and wanted to do seemed to widen, and she faltered and floundered, and her music seemed to disintegrate. I brought it to a close. Somehow in our music I found myself playing in rather an insensitive manner, musically aping the brash family style. Annabelle said there was a fairy that danced but then gradually fell asleep. I thought it was the very sensitive, imaginative side of herself that was being put to sleep by a rather too rational, matter-of-fact, no-nonsense approach to life. As she explored the instruments further, her face expressing keen delight at her kalimba glissandi, her fairy side timidly woke up out of its sleep. But at least her mother had been intuitive in feeling that music might be just what Annabelle needed even if she did ask "Is she worth teaching?" in front of the child.

The last example is Xena, the nine and a half year old daughter of a Czech mother and a Ghananian father. The parents were separated and the father had left the country when Xena was four. She studied the piano which she played musically with good rhythm. Xena started by exploring the instruments, playing a great number of them in a freely expressive way, working on different rhythms and timbres and preferring the larger percussion such as the gong, cymbal and 16" tom-tom. She decided that with these instruments she must have a Chinese story, possibly about an Emperor. She asked if she should tell it out loud but was told to think it and tell it to me afterwards. Her music was dynamic but well controlled and alternated between loud bursts on the tom-tom, cymbal and gong, a skipping theme on the xylophone, more thoughtful episodes on the melodica and some delicate passages on the bells. The story she told was as follows: The King came in and then the Princess. A Prince came and wanted to marry the Princess but the King said first he must kill a dragon. The Prince did this and returned with part of the dragon. Next he had to kill a sea serpent, and last---(pause)---a monster. He came back with part of the monster and went with the ladies-in-waiting to his house. Then he brought it to the king, who had a lot of princesses, and the Prince chose to marry the youngest.

It was understandable that Xena's first character was the father figure missing from her life and that she should manoeuvre a happy ending in which two people were united in marriage because she had not succeeded in keeping her own parents together. Perhaps if we had been able to work for longer she could have faced the depressive aspect of her inability to produce happy endings and have achieved the freedom from feeling that she could or should always do so.

Xena was very quiet and well-behaved over tea but when she told us the story of the book she was reading I could see little glints of fire so I was not surprised at the free aggression on the large percussion. However, I was surprised at how easily she could turn from these outbursts to her controlled skipping theme or tinkling on the bells. She, too, enjoyed the experience saying: "I like it here, I don't want to go!"

All these examples were from normal children in the sense that they were of normal or above-average intelligence, attended normal schools and had not had any kind of psychological treatment. And yet each one of them had their own personal difficulties and the music led them straight into making a symbolic statement of the condition in which they found themselves. It is easy to see how the therapy could proceed from there. Probably all but Tracey will work through their problems with the normal self-healing play and no outside help, to become well-adjusted adults. But their vulnerability is there and if there is playing to be done, either with a therapist or with their peers, this will be the work in the play.

With more disturbed children it might be some time before this freedom to play evolved and such frank statements of their difficulties emerged. For the disturbed children this creativity will be the preliminary aim of therapy rather than the starting place as with the normal child.

For ten years a colleague of mine, who does not want to be mentioned by name, has been giving a valuable preventive music therapy within a junior school setting. She found out from the teachers which children were under-achievers, withdrawn or hyperactive and took them out of the classroom, when it was convenient, in little groups of two to six. Occasionally, she took an individual child who showed evidence of more severe disturbance, on a one-to-one basis. Her method was to provide the setting of therapist, chairs and instruments and sit back and let the children play with them. She was available, if help or admiration or astonishment were sought, but she did not interfere or intrude in any way until near the end of the session when she might, if the children had not already asked for it, suggest the group come together in a musical story. I sat in on two days of this work and found it tremendously interesting. It was an admirable method of spotting both difficulties and disturbances and musical talent in a child. Here are some observations from my two day visit.

Some children showed an eager scientific interest in the instruments: How did they work? What could one do with them? With these children, guitar pegs were explored a great deal more than chords played. Others showed an instinctively artistic approach and expressed themselves freely on all instruments sometimes identifying themselves with a famous star player. Several Asian and one British child moved exotically as in a dance, quite unselfconsciously, while they played. Boys tended to act out their aggression while quiet, well-behaved girls played more gently but turned their aggression into malevolent and destructive fantasies usually concerning maternal symbols such as some caves which collapsed. Occasionally a child would get completely engrossed in creating a physical expression for his fantasy. One boy, who had quite a musical talent, put a tiny metallophone note up on the big xylophone and played them together with eager excitement probably exploring the possibility of parent and child coming together in some exciting connexion.

I expressed concern about Tom, who was very quiet at first, then very destructive to the xylophone notes, being apparently oblivious of the musical sound. He used the melodica only to make bike-horn and police siren sounds. His aggressive and sadistic fantasies seemed to make him unable to use his aggression in a normally constructive way of biting through a problem and getting to grips with it. It transpired that he had already been spotted and was having child guidance treatment.

Two nine year old boys, one Asian and one British, with heavy, ugly, quite unchildlike expressions seemed to get relief but no apparent pleasure from banging furiously and relentlessly on the drums without rhythm or pattern. My colleague said that a little girl had been the same but had worked through this phase to a kind of stunted curiosity in her play with a short span of concentration. It seemed that for these two the world was a joyless place and they were only able to pass on the kind of raw expression that they had experienced in it. I imagined that if this phase was not transcended they might later express these feelings in vandalism and destruction, but this is pure speculation.

My colleague said that sometimes the children were a bit excited after an uproarious session of twenty to thirty minutes but usually their teachers said they settled down well after their music sessions. I would like to look forward to a time when all primary schools had access to such preventive therapy.

Sometimes an analytical music therapist has child therapy thrust upon him when one of his mother out-patients is obliged to bring her offspring with her due to the lack of a childminder. In this case, as far as is possible, I ignore the child but give the mother time and space to attend to it as the mother may be testing the therapist to see if the child (symbolising a younger sibling) is preferred to herself. Some children, however, demand attention and then I give them a reasonable share before telling them that I want to talk to their mothers. I always include the child, if he shows any interest, in the music.

Here is an example of such a joint session. Meg could not find a child-minder for Nigel, who was nearly 5, so she brought him along with her to the session. She said that she had been terribly angry with him the day before: spanking him and telling him she would fetch the police and send him to a home. Later she had cuddled him and said it was not true. I asked what had happened. She said she had been hoovering all through the flat and Nigel had come along and split the hoover bag.

Nigel came forward forcefully and said he wanted us to play about trains; then he changed his mind and wanted us to play Monster. We did so. Nigel had bursts of aggression on the cymbal and drums while Meg was rather subdued on the xylophone. I played quite fiercely and once Nigel left the drums and came over to help me on the piano. When we heard the tape back, Nigel could not believe that those loud sounds were his; he went over by his mother and sucked his thumb. I said it was good to be near mother and have something to comfort him when he was frightened; he stopped sucking his thumb at once but started again at the next bang. Meg was amazed at this connexion. (Nigel's loud music coming out of the tape recorder became a kind of persecutory object, the music played being like a projection of bad parts of himself.) I also said that Nigel was sometimes a monster when he split the hoover bag and Mother was sometimes a monster when she spanked Nigel and said she was going to send him away when she did not mean it. Then I told Nigel that his Mother and I must talk but that he could play with any of the instruments as long as he was quiet. He explored the piano accordion only occasionally needing to be reminded of the decibel level. Later he came up and leant on my knee engaging my attention with urgent questions. I told him I thought he felt jealous when I took all Mother's attention and he quietly went back to his play. Later again he went out to the toilet alone. There were some strange noises and I asked Meg to go and see that he was not fiddling with anything electrical. "I couldn't reach the plug," he said stoutly when they returned. At the end of the session we played some music about his forthcoming school. Nigel did not play; he was exploring the pegs of the guitar. Meg played a bit louder than before and said she felt nervous about him going to school. Nigel spoke up saying he was not nervous about it at all. They functioned as a complimentary pair, Nigel was the bold extravert while Meg held all the weak feelings. When Nigel was with her, Meg was much quieter, allowing him to be their mouthpiece. When my colleagues returned and the pair left, it was Nigel that chirped, "Goodbye all!"

　　　In this brief essay there has not been time to discuss every aspect of analytical music therapy with children. Indeed, I do not consider myself experienced enough in this field to do so. In working with children, I am aware or their acute vulnerability. They offer you a tiny bud of creativity which can either grow and blossom and imbue them with a moving dignity and wholeness, or as easily be withered away. One must work with extreme delicacy.

　　　One can ask when does music therapy with children cease to be analytical and become regular music therapy? If one needs to split hairs in this way I would say it is when the use of words becomes wholly superfluous because of the child's lack of comprehension due to mental handicap. But even when there is no interpretation by the therapist because the child is already working and playing in a self-healing way, the analytical music therapist's exploratory approach will influence the way he helps to shape the movement of the therapy. With his assistance, the child will be led into controlling his environment in a creative way. As Winnicott (1971) wrote: "To control what is outside, one has to <u>do</u> things, not simply to think or to wish, and <u>doing things takes time</u>. Playing is doing" (p. 47). And analytical music therapy can provide an opportunity for such playing.

Essay   Twenty-Eight

Case Study: Couple Therapy

Fred is a sixty-six year-old tall, powerfully-built man with straight grey hair, dark eyes and glasses. He had retired as an engineer, and had suffered prior to this from agitated depression. At first he looked dejected and let his wife answer for him unless directly questioned. His attitude seemed to be that of a small child coming to his teacher with his mother. His agitation showed mostly in his clasping and unclasping his hands. He is a handsome man and gives the impression of supressing rage.

Inge is also tall, with straight brown hair done up on top of her head in a knot. She has a good figure, a pleasant unlined face and a bright and cheerful manner, though this felt to me like a veneer. She is a controlling sort of person, likes everything neat and tidy, answers for Fred in an apparent eagerness to be helpful and to protect him, but underneath this, one senses that she would be very threatened by any change in their relationship or mode of life. She was formerly a secretary.

Fred was referred to me by a Consultant Psychiatrist who was encouraged by the success we had with a previous agitated depressive patient of 62 who came for individual analytical music therapy. His consultant psychiatrist said that Fred first attended hospital at the age of forty-seven, with symptoms of endogenous agitated depression. He was then admitted three years later for three weeks, six years later for seven weeks and in the next year for ten weeks. In between he regularly attended the out-patients' clinic. The present episode had lasted for two years.

For four months, at the end of the first year, a female clinical psychologist gave Fred relaxation and concentration training and a focus on leisure interests. For the next year the principal clinical psychologist tried to improve his motivation via a cognitive approach, and in his final report stated that he felt that the marital relationship had improved, but that there was little more that could be achieved with this approach. (Fred said that the psychologist had persuaded him to drive his car again and this had been very important to him). Fred was referred to me 8 months later by the consulting psychiatrist.

It was not my original intention to take both of them on as a couple, but, as at first I only had a fortnightly vacancy, I thought that perhaps this could be helpful for several reasons: they would have the opportunity of carrying on the therapy attitudes in between sessions and in holidays; each could see alternative and possibly more fruitful ways of interacting with the other; the therapist could see the main influence that each one was under for 167 hours a week and, if necessary, try to promote helpful changes; Fred and Inge would have the opportunity to grow and develop together, instead of one getting left behind and then being dispensed with, as frequently happens when one of a couple is having therapy; the therapist could validate their relationship as a potential force for good, intrapersonally, interpersonally and in society; the therapist could validate them each as unique individuals (this is especially valuable for the average wife) not just in their marital roles; the therapist could open up areas which the couple had not discussed previously; couples who have become totally "Adult" and "Parental" (as in the Transactional Analysis sense) could perhaps also learn to play together; and there would be the opportunity to work with, and explore, the subtle emotional nuances of the couple at various levels.

When we first started I thought it could be helpful for them both to answer the Beck Depression Inventory, which consists of 21 questions all with 4 possible graded answers on such subjects as self-image, level of depression, sexual appetite, hunger, sleep and so on. The higher the score the more depressed the patient. Throughout the period of treatment their scores were as follows (out of a possible maximum of 84):

	Fred	Inge
January 1988	31	6.5
July 1988	26	12
September 1988	22	6
November 1988	20	7.5
March 1989	22	10

It was significant that apart from the last score, which was affected by their anxiety about being able to do the tasks, as Fred became less depressed, Inge became more depressed.

At first Fred was resistant to any attempt at history-taking. But he agreed to answer this questionnaire, during which it came out that he felt very suicidal and was eyeing the sharp knife in the kitchen with a thought of slashing his wrists. Inge collapsed in tears as she had not realised that he felt like that. Their first music was an improvisation on how they felt. Fred had the 16" drum, xylophone, cymbal and gong, and Inge had another drum and a glockenspiel. Their music, though tentative at first, became robust and rhythmic. However, it somehow always produced in my piano improvisation a level of banality of which I was ashamed but could not alter. It was clear that their music afforded both of them a much-needed outlet for self-expression. I asked Fred to give us a loud cymbal clash as our signal to finish. Throughout our working period I treated him as the head of the family, trying to ease him out of the "Woman-on-Top" position, as his original attitude was very much that of a sulky four-year-old child who has everything done for him but has no status in the family. Inge spoilt him and nagged him. She felt very angry that he got so behind with the gardening and home maintenance jobs that normal husbands in suburban homes take upon themselves. Fred felt only faintly guilty about this but mostly his attitude appeared to be a mixture of triumphant smugness and brooding sulleness. The idea that there could be any way round this stalemate seemed unacceptable to both of them. As they were not cripplingly short of money I asked if they had thought of hiring a lad for a weekend to cope with the backlog. Fred could not think of letting someone else do his jobs. It seemed that this cold war was entirely necessary to both of them. Internally Fred mourned for his life with working men, and Inge resented him sitting like an immovable object intruding into the time and space of her queendom.

As depression is often based on anger bound by guilt, I devised some exercises to express aggression in a non-threatening way on two 16" tom-toms. Each of them had to play on his own drum then reach over and bang on the other's drum. First the other had to reply, "NO" and then, when Fred gave the signal, to say "Yes" and afterwards share feedback. When Inge poached on to Fred's drum and he said, "No!" he stared fixedly at her for some time as if wondering: "Is it going to be accepted or will she burst into tears?" At home this was her answer to any attempt on his part to alter any of her established ways. When Fred mentioned that a retired friend was having cookery lessons Inge said she would go mad if he came into her kitchen.

In the fourth session, two weeks later, Fred reported seeing two boys fighting while he was mowing the lawn, and going over and stopping them. He then remembered his mother giving him boxing gloves and then taking them away when he and his little brother began sparring. He said he was never angry, although to me he looked as if he were seething with an anger that could find no possible outlet. At this time it showed only verbally in the occasional snide remark. For example, when Inge said that as an only child she was very self-willed and her mother had said she always managed to get her own way, Fred said darkly and without humour, "You still do!" She ignored this.

When they came on their 36th wedding anniversary he muttered grimly that it was not like it used to be 36 years ago. From the questionnaire it emerged that they were not sexually active though they still slept in a double bed. There was obviously a lot of tension in this area but I did not feel that they were ready to speak about this problem. It crossed my mind that Inge might have a lover.

In the eighth session, we had three drums and my poaching on to their drums was to represent an intrusion into their marriage or a stimulus. Their "NO" response was rather restrained but their "YES" was gracious and inviting.

These exercises were alternated with "Cave Mouth" and "Mountain Climb" visualisations with improvised music. Assagioli (1965), creator of Psychosynthesis, used these techniques and others as diagnostic tools. The couple responded readily and vividly to visualisation with music, and I felt it would give them a release from the frustrating prisons of their present daily existence, promote a more fruitful interaction with the unconscious, and give Fred especially, an area of creativity and action that his present state denied him.

We also improvised on "Holiday," which they both used for reminiscence, and the reflection on their lives between the ages of 0 and 30 (curiously both only had memories from the age of 18), and 30 to 66, which brought up their happy holidays abroad (which Fred used to organise) and the old age and death of both their parents.

In the eleventh session, we did a musical acting scene. Two people were to meet, chat together, find that they disagreed quite vehemently, argue, then cool down and part. When Fred and I did this in music his physical response was quite striking. His face went into a snarl showing his teeth, his whole body squirmed but his drumming expressed very little. However, Inge and I were able to be quite sharp with one another. Repeating the exercise with Fred, having told him how he looked and sounded, he was able to be more forceful on the drum and more relaxed in his body. After this, for the first time, Inge began to cry very modestly, wiping every tear meticulously with her handkerchief. She gave vent to very despairing feelings: "What's the use of anything? There is so much to do in the house and garden and he just sits there like a lump." She was afraid to tell him what she felt for fear of making him worse. He was afraid to speak to her as she cried at the slightest thing. She could not bear to see him all tense and clutching his hands. As previously she had maintained that she was never depressed and always busy with two jobs at once, I felt that sharing these despairing feelings could be a helpful gain in truth with a subsequent access of the energy which had kept these feelings suppressed.

At the end of this session we did the first of the musical visualisations on "Creating My Room," "My Garden," and "My Village." Interestingly enough, in Inge's series there were animals, tropical fish, swans and ducks. Her animal nature, being denied both sex and normal relaxation, was begging to be considered. Fred visualised a swimming pool, light and brilliantly coloured flowers and football games. This gave me a clue as to what activities he might become involved in later, and the fact that he would like to experience strong feelings as a normal part of his life. In response to Fred's interest in swimming Inge said that she hated water.

In certain ways the couple were very closely attuned to each other. To see what would happen in a physically "Man-on-Top" situation, one day I brought some records of dance music which they had spoken about, and they danced most beautifully together with Fred taking a definite lead and Inge following, their bodies in close and perfect physical harmony. Another day we did the "Tapping Game" in which one person goes out and has to come in and perform an act pre-decided by the others in the room; the only clue they get is the tapping by their partner or someone else in the room, loud for "on the trail" and soft or silence for "wrong direction." Their tuning to each other verged on the extra-sensory as without hesitation each in turn found their way to carrying out the secret act with their partner doing the tapping. Perhaps they were too closely attuned and vulnerable to each other's negative signals and that was why Fred could not function at home as he did in the session where he was more in tune with my belief in him as a separate and capable person.

In the thirteenth session, Inge came alone, distraught. Fred had refused to get out of bed. She wept and said, "It is all too much, I have to do everything and we never do anything nice together." They had had a quarrel because she had felt obliged to mow the lawn with the heavy motor mower. Then, having been invited out to lunch and a film, and feeling guilty about leaving Fred, she had banged a door in fury and he had woken with a start thinking it was an electrical fault. As Inge reiterated that she was not the patient, we did no music, which she believed to be the therapy, being unaware of the psychotherapeutic aspect of our verbal exchange. I tried to ring Fred at once but gave up after waiting in vain for quarter of an hour for our hospital operator to answer. When I later spoke to Fred on the phone he was cheerful and apologetic. I said that it was when one felt really bad that the therapy was most useful. In the next session we explored feelings about "Going" and "Not Going." I explained that we were working with energies and they might find themselves getting quite irritable until they had learnt to use these energies constructively.

There was a lot of guilt floating about. Inge's unconscious death-wish for Fred made it impossible for her to adapt to the unhappy circumstance of his illness by allowing herself any pleasure. Also her frantic need to control, made her a slave to the house and garden and hairdresser, and to respond negatively and destructively in our sessions to Fred's little sparks of enthusiasm for cooking, cycling, swimming, football, a weekend break away, and his stamp collection.

In sessions 26 and 39, I tackled her on this, pointing out the difference between nagging someone to make them do what you wanted, and encouraging them when they showed some enthusiasm for something themselves. In session 39, she became quite hysterical, weeping and screaming, "You don't have him 24 hours a day, he never says he wants to do ANYTHING! I can't stand it any more, if I had anywhere to go I'd run away!" I asked Fred if he thought she might leave him and he said, "Yes, sometimes." To illustrate my point Fred said he had felt that he could, as the head of the household, fill in the Electoral Roll form but found that Inge had already done it.

In some ways Fred's illness fulfilled an unused early maternal instinct in Inge. Through it she could experience the total power that the mother has over an infant. But real motherhood compels the mother to adapt herself gradually to the child's growing independence and self-determination. Inge had not had to learn that. In another way Fred's sitting at home represented a frightened baby part of herself being kept from terrors such as floods, storms, and terrorist attacks which she often spoke about. The fact that Fred, in his depressed and apathetic state, fulfilled a meaningful, though unconscious, function for Inge, was a factor in the couple wanting to preserve the status quo, as it at least gave Fred a kind of usefulness and meaning, albeit pathological, whereas the life of retirement seemed utterly meaningless to him. It also meant that Inge could split off this anxious little part of herself and project it on to Fred, and then see herself only as a normal, busy and cheerful person.

During all this time their music was vigorous and rhythmic and Fred became increasingly musically inventive. They came into the sessions eagerly but Inge wanted to make therapy a social occasion and competed with Fred conversationally for my attention. From session 31, I let Fred lead the sessions. In 31, he wanted to talk, in 32 to relax to music, in 33 to improvise to "Shopping." In 31 Fred said he was afraid that he had Alzheimer's Disease. I said the fear hid a wish for an excuse to live blamelessly like an infant. I told him to tell the Consultant and wrote to him myself. Inge had by now actually been out to lunch alone, but Fred had made her feel guilty by only eating a banana.

In session 36, he came in looking pale and ill. The Consultant had said there were no signs of Alzheimer's Disease. In 38, they came in strangely excited. Inge was to have a cataract operation and be away for a week. Now that she was not going to enjoy herself, she felt sure Fred could cope alone for a week. Fred said rather hopefully that last time she was ill away he ate his supper in a cafe. Inge said she would fill the freezer for him. (Mother again!) Inge talked, almost hopefully, about dying. Fred felt that life had become one routine for him with breaks for dentist, hairdresser and therapy. I felt this as the Kiss of Death for our work and started once more to direct the sessions myself.

In sessions 40 and 41, they each did a musical "Family Sculpture." They became very lively with vivid memories. Later Fred remembered that his brother had had a secret early breakdown and he phoned him for the first time in years. Family sculpture is a technique that I learnt in the Institute of Group Analysis and later adapted to include music. The client places instruments of his choice in positions to indicate his emotional distances from his family members. We wanted to reveal the patterns of childhood. He then describes how he felt about each family member and they improvise duets, she (or the therapist) in the role of each member in turn. After feedback, the partner tells what she, as family member, felt about each emotional and geographical placing. The client regards the pattern of instruments and decides if he would like to move anyone. It is a strangely powerful technique.

In session 43, I decided to crack the whip. The time of my retirement was approaching and despite our lively sessions, their homelife was still so stagnant that I felt it necessary to try to heal the split between these states. In life there are life-preserving routines and deadening sleep-producing routines. I felt that this couple had a mutually collusive conspiracy to remain in one of the latter. I rang the principal clinical psychologist who had felt the same. The vortex of stagnation alarmed me as one of our patients had stayed in a depression for 18 ongoing years. I told the couple that our department had a waiting list and unless they personally could do the tasks appointed during the next seven sessions they must leave. Each week each was to do a self-chosen enjoyable "ego" task and Fred was also to choose a duty to do. We played stormy music about this plan and Fred was given a notebook to record their progress because in an exercise about work he had said he had enjoyed taking the minutes at meetings. Fred, with prompting, chose to fill in his income tax form for his duty, and to go to the pub for his ego task, then he looked miserable and said no, he wouldn't enjoy it. Inge suggested that he watch football instead, and he agreed.

It became the pattern that they could not think of ego tasks unless their partner suggested them. (Privately I translated this sexually into "I cannot have sex unless my partner initiates it and I cannot masturbate in our double bed"). They came to session 44 tense and glum. Fred had looked at his tax form but not completed it. However, both ego tasks had been done and enjoyed. As Fred had totally ignored their wedding anniversary Inge bought herself a new needlework box and rung her friend in South Africa at some length without guilt. After our music, Fred said reparatively that he was making real melodies. And he was.

By session 46, the routine of the tasks was well established, the expectant mood had come back as all tasks were done, the "duty" ones sometimes minimally but the "ego" ones were producing spin-offs. Inge brought me flowers from their garden but kept bleating,"Fred only does what I say." I began to realise that there could be an element of jealousy and of fear of loss of control. In the same session, each of us in turn danced our "Inner Music" while the two others accompanied it. Inge's dance was graceful and Fred danced in a Polynesian style, wiggling his posterior at us provocatively. For the first time Inge came out with a whole-hearted compliment. "Fred used to be a lovely dancer." He denied this but from his smile we could see he was pleased.

I realise that I have said very little about the couple's actual music. From the beginning their music was energetic and rather deadeningly rhythmic. Fred favoured a longish improvisation. Inge would beseech him, non-verbally, to stop three-quarters of the way through, but for once Fred was "Man-on-Top" and was not going to terminate before he chose to do so. The music revealed them as being sustainers rather than innovators. Perseverance was their virtue. As Fred, especially, found it threatening to express aggression or even assertion verbally, the music became a reliable container for his rage and rebellion. It always reduced his agitation. But it also could express delight and a playful approach which began to verge on the musically creative.

From session 47 onward, Inge started to rebel against the ego tasks, preferring to make an effort to do something enjoyable involving Fred. She took him shopping to the West End and later to the local

Garden Centre. I reminded her that I had suggested the ego tasks on the basis of her saying that she was so unhappy that she wanted to run away. But at least they had helped to give her a clearer feeling of direction. In answer to her repeated frantic, "When will he be better?" I felt that they were strong enough now for me to say that no one knew, we could only work at each day as it came; some depressions lasted days, one patient was still depressed after eighteen years. I thought it was a risk telling them this but nevertheless I felt intuitively that for them it was right. The reaction to it was a great leap forward. During the next week they visited Kew Gardens at Fred's (first) suggestion, went to a pub where Fred had his first pint of beer since retirement, and almost completed the dreaded income tax form. In the last improvisation before the completion of this paper, "Playing for Fun," Fred put tremendous energy into his music with a cheeky drummed "dum dada dum dum--pom pom" motif, echoed on the piano. It seemed that he was giving us courage to believe that he was by no means such a hopeless case.

This was a stubborn and difficult case, and I believed that the couple's consolidation of their growth and development evinced in the sessions would take much longer than the time available for our work. For Inge, Fred represented unconsciously both her dependent and submissive child and a frightened agoraphobic part of herself. Therefore she was very threatened by any voiced enthusiasm or interest on his part, discouraged it promptly and then denied its existence. As Fred was unable to be affirmative still, even less aggressive, his reaction to this was rebellious apathy punctuated by the odd snide remark. I think my ability not to be black-mailed by Inge's hysteria at mild criticism, or Fred's intense agitation when asked to choose an ego task, gave each a model for being a bit firmer in daring to speak to the other. Several times during reminiscences Inge reported being surprised to hear Fred relate something about his past. For example she was amazed to hear that his father beat him when he was naughty. "Fred naughty? I can't believe it!" she said. However, she never surprised him in that way.

Our exploration of the history of the pair as a couple helped their dyadic group image through their reminiscences of the good holidays Fred organised and their support of their old parents. Their personal identities seemed to be totally group-oriented. Fred had no activities at home to express his individuality, he was either Inge's servant or nothing. He could only be something through his male peer group. The ego tasks were an antidote to this. Inge also functioned as she thought wives should and did, rather than responding sensitively and creatively to Fred's needs of the moment and her own wishes for growth and development personally. For example, she continued to serve him huge three course-dinners when he was overweight from inactivity and drugs, saying, "My mother always cooked a good dinner for father and I." If he did not make a clean plate, she wept. Fred could complain about this in the session, trusting me to contain Inge's emotional reaction, but not yet at home. His aggressive and playful feelings had an increasingly free outlet in his music but the transition from musical expression to verbal would have had to take more time. Furthermore I felt that Inge's brittle but fragile ability to cope emotionally could easily crumble disasterously if rigorous methods of confrontation were employed. And that could mean his re-admission to hospital.

Writing this in April, the therapy was due to terminate in five months, when I retired from institutional work. During that time I had hoped to help them to learn how to disagree more constructively, and how to evoke their Homo Ludens aspect through musical games, creative experiences with their bodies and dancing. I hoped that this might invalidate Fred's remark that their lives were, "All work and no play."

After fifteen and a half months of music therapy Inge was increasingly able to accept some of her own depressive feelings thus using less energy on defending herself against them. She felt more able to see friends and to set goals for herself and Fred (though I doubt whether he was yet included in the planning of them). She was also a little more inclined to try to make the best of the present rather than feeling that nothing could be achieved until Fred was better. She said that her aims for the future were to help housebound old people and to enjoy more of their successful holidays abroad again.

Fred showed much more initiative verbally and musically in the sessions. His posture was more upright and his self-image somewhat improved. He was beginning to take real pleasure in improvising music, to see himself as a member of a musical family and even entertain a faint wish to learn to play tunes in the future. He realised that he needed to get back into his peer group and this was to be achieved by joining his firm's retirement club at a later date. He said he also would like to be a volunteer driver for hospital patients when he felt strong enough. Altogether I felt that the work showed that music therapy can offer a useful and multi-faceted approach to couple therapy but with an older couple there needs to be a much longer time for readjustment with support and understanding. I was sorry that in this I had to let them down.

Essay Twenty-Nine

Intertherapy

Intertherapy is the name given to the second part of the orientation training for analytic music therapists. The first part of the training is the experience of the trainee as being the client of a trained analytical music therapist. During this part the trainee learns something about what a therapist is and does and tries to avoid doing. He begins to explore his own inner life with the aid of shared music and words and, hopefully, he will put some trust in the work that he and his therapist do together. He will probably begin to understand something of the power of improvised music to express his own feelings in contrast to playing those of a composer. He will surely also have some experiences which will enable him to empathise more closely with his clients as they trace some of their emotional roots back into their earliest years. In this way he will come to understand their woundedness and their fears about the repetition of that pain. But he will also begin to expand and experience the joy of his shared and accepted expression in the musical dyad, in the verbal dialogues with his therapist and perhaps also just in their mutuality of being.

It is essential that someone aiming at practicing AMT should have this experience as a client with someone who is trained in AMT, because only this will help him towards an understanding of his own patients and the right sensitivity and care in the therapeutic use of this powerful art form. It is here, too, that he learns about his own vulnerability through music and the way it can lead him to preverbal memories, symbolic images and emotions that he never realised he had.

If such powerful experiences were to arise for the first time when he was acting as therapist, he would be likely to lose his holding power completely and cease, at least temporarily, to be of therapeutic use to the patient. Or he might be tempted to leave his devotion to the patient in the improvisation and only explore his own inner journey which would be most ill-advised. This, of course, would be quite different from the therapeutic split-awareness of his patient's music; and the emotions and sensations that her music's unexpressed feelings were creating in him. In this case he is only using himself and his inner awareness as a kind of instrument for echoing the depths of her repressed or suppressed feelings.

Regarding the dialogue in the therapy, where a trainee has had no experience of longer-term analytical psychotherapy of once weekly or more, he may need anything from 20-120 AMT sessions before he feels ready to start the Intertherapy. However, most trainees in this position have gone on to have some analytical psychotherapy when they have started work after the training and found this helpful.

Music therapy training courses differ in their provision of collegial supervision for course members in the first year of their practice. There are also differences of opinion as to what supervision is. Some young musicians are bogged down by a rather Oedipal view of a supervisor as a particularly evil and repressive kind of conductor-parent who is going to stop them from discovering their own best way to work. I was lucky enough to be directed to the Jungian analytic supervisor who wrote the introduction to this book. He was very helpful to me over eleven years at a time when there were no local analytical music therapists to whom I could turn, although not a trained musician he not infrequently pointed something out in the taped improvisations that I had missed. Mind you I did not always see it in this way, and now and then raged at him for not being the applauding audience I had come to expect, need and appreciate from my early performing days. However, the astringency did me good when I was not feeling too stressed. On those days the sudden appearance through the balcony window of a large fluffy ginger cat walking round his indoor tree was pacifying to my inner music.

The original Intertherapy in which I was therapist to Peter Wright and patient to Marjorie Wardle who was patient to Peter, was a learning and research enterprise rolled into one. We had no observing supervisor as the odd men out used the time to write up their notes; some of mine were legible enough for use in later publication. As we were all equally inexperienced we preferred to make our own discoveries as best as we could, but occasionally the listener, after having finished with her notes, would make a comment afterwards, behaving in some sort of supervisory role.

At the time we felt that it was not fair to subject our patients to experimental techniques that we had not experienced for ourselves.

If there were any snags or dangers we would be willing to encounter them ourselves first, before we decided whether these were suitable techniques to be used with the emotionally disturbed. Another matter was that nearly all our patients were quite heavily medicated, and even if we had tried these techniques on the them first, we would hardly have had any proper idea of the full impact of such work if we had not let some relatively adequately functioning healthy, undrugged people, who could give some articulate feedback, undergo this experimental trial. Actually I was on some medication and had had personal experience of the incapaciting effect of some of the side effects of the various fashionable drugs. But this was quite useful,too.

After the initial one-to-one AMT, the two trainees take it in turns to be therapist and patient, and the trained analytical music therapists acts only as observer/supervisor. This is the "Intertherapy" component of the training. As far as possible, the observing supervisor's brief is to allow the therapy to happen. The trainee therapist must be enabled to find his own style, to make contact with the "patient" in his individual way and to feel comfortable in this role. But not too comfortable. There are anyway so many discomforts in the practice of therapy that one does not want to add to them by engendering a sense of unease and self-consciousness in the trainees. So the observer/supervisor allows the "therapist" to be the therapist and the "patient" to be the patient. His presence should be easily forgotten and what remains of it should help the "therapist" to internalise a helpful observer. It is part of being a therapist to experience this benign split into the acting and watching parts of being. One could say that the one part acts in the therapy and the other part writes the notes afterwards. The "patient" in this situation will want to preserve a split awareness of his colleague's techniques as well as his own needs and feelings.

The supervisor empathically feels himself into the inner music of the therapeutic couple, and remains observant and silent for as long as he can. While the therapy is moving, even stammering, silent or raging, he can leave them to themselves and take up any points afterwards. At first he may take over the time-keeping function for the therapists but later he will let them take back this responsibility as they progress. (Trainee therapists are usually so excited about their new roles that they are appalling time-keepers and the supervisor is well advised to watch the time even when they are supposed to be time-keeping for themselves, or he may find that he has run well into the next session and the day's work is sliding into the dinner hour).

As regards time, the whole Intertherapy session should be planned for a good two hours. The trainee's sessions last about half an hour each, and the supervisor may only have a therapeutic discussion at the end of the sessions, or he may want to give some hints on technique and theory at the beginning as well. Before the Intertherapy finishes, it is advisable to let the trainees have one or more whole-hour sessions each, to get the feeling of this timespan. This is usually a great relief which gives a feeling of freedom and relaxation that will help the trainees to look forward to their forthcoming professional sessions. However, they will probably realise that there was also value in concentrating the work into half an hour, in that they will then know that a surprising amount of work can be done in a short space of time when necessary. Genuine hospitalised patients, on the whole, need longer for tuning as they often do not really move until the last quarter of an hour. My supervisor once suggested taking sessions of an hour and a half but the therapist also has to be able to stand this.

In AMT there are three kinds of language to observe: verbal language, body language and the language of music. It would be rather difficult for a trainee to give a picture of all three later on to a supervisor absent from the session. I have found that the trainee therapist needs to have immediate help with his blind spots in the initial stages of the work. Later on when he starts work, his supervisor will have to manage from a recording of the music together with verbal feedback. Some students are good at picking up points from one language, others at another but usually one will be left out and need to be emphasised a little more.

Having lived abroad where I did not at first know the language, and having shared my life with plants, babies and animals, I find that I am keenly attentive to body language and voice tone. This often escapes a trainee who can be dazzled by a particularly articulate trainee patient. Sometimes these languages complement and sometimes contradict one another. One must also be sensitive to double messages. The aggressive music may be the positive of a negative, inhibited body language, accompanied by measured and controlled speech in defensively flat tones. Or a vital verbal flow and free body language may accompany a stunted musical language.

As an example, a suicidal young mother had an inert body language, chaotic torrents of verbal flow and frenzied aggression on the instruments at the beginning of her therapy. At the end of the work, which was shared in group therapy later on, some of that musical aggression had turned into firm speech, decisive action and measured, rather feeble music-making, which coincided with a negative transference.

As another example: a young lawyer whose speech was fairly shallow and evasive, and whose body language seemed to indicate a desire to escape, had the most searching, powerful, expressive and direct vocal musical expression. I was not able to follow this up for many sessions as he did, indeed, escape. I would have been most interested to watch any redistribution or benign contagion from this fine musical expression. All three languages offer valuable gates to the understanding of a person. None should be ignored.

To go back to the Intertherapy sessions, the most obvious point for interjection by the supervisor is the point at which the title for the improvisation is decided. This title may focus the therapy in a vital direction for the work, or it may turn away from this important aim and make the music into a defensive and vapid note-patting. It is here that the trainee therapist could use some help, and the supervisor may break in to ask, "May I make a suggestion?" and if the couple agrees he will let them have the benefit of his experience in choosing a title.

For example, one trainee patient was telling how another girl had entered her and her fiance's life. Instead of exploring the existing feelings about this, the trainee therapist immediately picked on a title of pious hope or magical solution in "Trios that work." Now this could have been a worthy aim but it was hardly an exploration of the immediate situation. I let them play this as it seemed to be right to allow them to continue at the time, their collusion in avoiding the deeper issues having given them a certain closeness. But later we looked at the possibility that there could have been a suppressed fear of abandonment masking jealousy, which was also heavily defended against by both the trainees who were rather narrowly religious.

Neither of them had had any previous therapy and both were averse to admitting even the possibility of entertaining any such ignoble suppositions.

Another time the trainee patient started her session by saying that she was angry about coming that evening, angry about money. Her trainee therapist suggested that they should play a palliative "Going Home" but I suggested that she should play "Getting What I Want," as I felt that it led to where the feeling of angry deprivation was. The music really expressed the need and the patient was left feeling that she wanted to cry and cry and cry in sheer frustration of her desires.

Some motivated, less-defended patients are adept at choosing revealing titles that will forward the work, but most need to be led in the right direction, at least towards the beginning. Later on the therapist will feel more sure of himself in the role and possibly the "patient" will be more certain of where he wants to go. However, in the initial sessions the supervisor's choice can be usefully educative. When the supervisor thinks the pair would benefit from a guiding interjection, but feels that this might destroy something creative that is happening in the relationship at that moment, he will make a note of it and talk about it later.

This brings us to the question of the supervisor taking notes. In this role I have found it absolutely necessary to make quick notes of points that come up in the Intertherapy sessions. Things as different as a repeated word accompanied by a gesture, the use of instruments and beater when the music is not being played, or a musical reaction to the therapist's sforzando, cannot always easily be recalled by the time the second therapy has taken place and the supervisor has a point or two of his own to remember to tell them. It is hard to be as receptive as possible and at the same time to hang on to all these small points. Certainly some trainees have been a bit paranoid about their supervisor's note-taking at first but when it was realised that every jotting was not so much a bad mark as a helpful suggestion or even the odd congratulation, then it was usually tolerated with equanimity.

It has been said in protest that if you take notes you lose something said, but things kept in the mind tend to gather associations and then the mind will screen out just as much. No one but an eidetic memory phenomenon is totally receptive. When the thinking person comes to recall, there has almost always been some unconscious editing out. The trainees must simply have trust in their "good-enough" supervisor and put all thoughts of omniscient parent figures away together with childish omnipotence.

Still on the subject of notes, it is interesting to discover at what point the supervisor's notes turn to doodling, because when the little men and cats and houses in the mountains start appearing in the notebook I have usually found that there was something going dead in the training therapy. It seems to take the place of the supervisory therapist getting bored and starting to yawn. That is often the time when the trainee patient is sitting on some material that she ought to be talking about and is unconsciously refusing to do any honest work.

I have written at length about the necessity for the supervisor's sensitivity, tact and empathy towards the therapeutic couple but some thought must be given to his own feelings in this strange situation, and his reaction to them. He must be aware that the aim of the other two members of the trio is to get rid of him and make him superfluous, he is in the role of the middle-aged parent who is expendable. He is operating, too, as the excluded third party in a triangle. First of all this can stir up feelings from earlier periods in his life when he was an excluded third party, possibly in a trio of mother and father against him, or mother and sister against him. This may arouse in him an impulse to interject at all costs, or it may cause his interest in the intimate scene revealed before him to die mysteriously away. If he understands these possibilities he will be able to withstand the feelings better and to act from this understanding rather than from blind impulse.

Another matter that can bear thought is that he will remain receptive to sometimes extremely emotional words and music for longer periods than would be normal for a therapist, acting as a container, without (if you exclude his brief note-taking) any opportunity for focussed creativity at all. This can create a situation where when he is allowed to speak, either he finds that there is nothing there, or it bursts out of him in an overwhelming explosion rather than a therapeutic communication. What can he do about it? He can, first of all, be aware of it, and secondly he can see that the rest of his day contains some opportunites for focussed creativity: writing and speaking and performing music would be excellent antidotes. Failing that---one is left with the gnomes and cats. Any more heavily receptive or passive activities would be less useful. These are my experiences but people differ.

So far the supervisor has been only a supervisor but towards the end of the Intertherapy things can change. He may need to give both trainees a model for an alternative way for a therapist to handle his patient. One way is to perhaps do a little therapy with the trainees in their patient roles while all three are sitting round equidistant after the therapy sessions. Another is to be a therapist to the trainees in their therapist roles, helping them to express their feelings and thoughts about the sessions. It sounds rather confusing, but in fact it can work out quite smoothly and naturally when the supervisor is flexible. One does not invariably have to speak in all four roles. Trainees at first tend to expect a judgment of their performance as therapist and patient, and are surprised to find themselves encouraged to produce some thoughts and feelings on which to base their own judgements, if indeed judgements there must be. Perhaps we should say reflections.

What sort of thing should a supervisor look out for? He will notice the therapist's attitude towards the patient: Is he warm or cold, empathetic rather than sympathetic? Does he dominate the verbal dialogue or is he able to be receptive but enabling? What kind of body messages is he giving? Is he getting at the music behind the words? What is going on between the pair? Shall he let them struggle through a sticky patch and find their own way, or break in before they waste any more time? Is the therapist modelling himself on a teacher, priest, parent or the supervisor who gave him his earlier individual session, or is he managing to find his own style? Is the therapist giving reassurance in a way that does not allow the patient to ventilate her deeper anxieties? Is he finding magical solutions in the way of good advice or palliative improvisation titles aimed only at "kissing it better" rather than allowing the situation as it is, or seems to be, to be fully explored? Is he criticising the patient for expressing negative feelings? Is he able to bring out feelings that the patient is near to but not yet aware of? Does the patient feel controlled or merely held? Can he change with the patient's mood in the music or does he get lost playing a concerto and giving himself a bit of therapy? Does he pick up unconscious feelings? (It usually takes some time to do this with confidence). Does the music take the supervisor along with it? If it does it always means that something real and good is happening.

Each supervisor will develop his own style of note-taking but one or two ideas of mine may be helpful. I write my own thoughts, questions and comments in square brackets, and subject headings, significant gestures and phrases outside. In this way I can easily pick out what I want to say afterwards. Improvisation titles I always underline (or at least I always mean to underline); this makes them stand out so that one can easily skim through one's notebook and see the direction that the therapy has taken to date. If the supervisor does not write shorthand it can be helpful to devise short forms for such recurring words as mother, father, died, feelings, countertransference, sex, sister, brother, lover, husband, wife and so on.

Some students comment on how hard it is to switch from the patient role (and sometimes there are tears which are hard to stanch) to the therapist role; it is somewhat easier the other way round. But always I am amazed at how well students do this. I recall most vividly one professor psychiatrist musician hunched up in his chair sobbing like a seven year old as the "patient," and the next minute sitting upright with his best chairside manner and showing real concern for the erstwhile therapist now patient.

It is not a bad idea for a student to realise that he is capable of this change of role, for as a working therapist he will be vulnerable to life's bruises outside therapy and have to walk into the workroom and put his own troubles behind him until his working day is finished. Until he has tried it he will not realise his strength in focussing his mind firmly in one direction towards another human being in trouble.

Acting as a supervisor can be a real help towards making a therapist take a long, hard look at his own work. He can find that he is picking out some of his own worst faults in the therapist and they may come to meet him when he goes back to his own patients. He may also find the supervisor part of himself sitting on his own shoulder and asking, "What do you think you are doing now?" at awkward moments. But if he survives, it can be most salutory.

It is quite important to those students who are not already doing some practical work in a psychiatric ward or hospital, that the supervisor should warn the trainees that their real life patients are most unlikely to show anything like the range and depth of expression that they, as qualified music therapists and musicians, have done. Far from the danger being that a great explosion from the unconscious will express itself in sound and blow the patient's brains out (as some members of the audiences of talks that we gave earlier on seemed to fear) the greatest danger in reality seems to be that absolutely nothing will happen over and over again, so that anything that takes place above this level is a bonus for both patient and therapist. One must, of course, expect a different level of excitement in medicated and unmedicated patients, and one must also realise that levels of expressed emotion considered quite normal in certain cultures would have psychiatrists in this country reaching for some very heavy medication. For example, in the twenty years that I have worked in hospital I have seldom worked with a patient who cried more than a few trickling tears, but in the Intertherapy I have experienced real sobbing that shook the whole body not once but many times. There has been vocal sexual expression so strong in a non-medicated client that the group case discussion leader rushed to turn the cassette recorder's volume down in case his children and womenfolk upstairs would think that their father's group had degenerated into a saturnalian orgy.

Every therapist has his own ideas and wants to remain creative; so when the time of the formal Intertherapy is over, it has been helpful to some therapists to form an Intertherapy of colleagues both for working through current problems and dreams (I have not found a better therapy for dreams) and also for developing new techniques which are always best experimented with on one's peers who can give some searching feedback. One of the reasons for continuing on an informal basis among colleagues is that the work with drugged hospitalised or out-patients will tend to make the therapist forget what a potentially powerful medium AMT can be.

Another frequent result of the work in Intertherapy is the freer power of musical expression which the students so often gain. This carries over into their formal musical performance and gives greater spontaneity and flexibility of expression.

The trainee who has satisfactorily expressed his own triumph or rage on the drums with a musical holding from his therapist, can better ally himself with Beethovenian sforzandi in a violin or piano sonata. If he has managed to find some notes to clothe his own deepest sadness and highest joy he can better feel his way into some of the haunting melodies of Brahms. He has released his own springs of expression and creativity at a deep level and will no longer be satisfied with a cosmetic interpretation of the music of men and women who were able to feel as deeply and passionately as himself.

Intertherapy is a discipline with many discomforts and inconveniences. It can be extremely frustrating but it can also be a valuable path of development for the trainee in AMT. With this short orientation training he will be aware that he has just started on a life's work in a certain direction, there is no rubber stamp on him saying that he knows it all. Also the short time available ensures that the work proceeds step by step, for, as it says in the Tao Te Ching: "Great carving is not done by hacking."

Essay Thirty

Ending The Session Or Treatment

The beginning and ending of the analytical music therapy session will probably mark the start and finish of a different kind of relationship from those the patient will have experienced elsewhere. Within this time-space the patient can rely on almost total and constant attention from her therapist for the purpose of helping her in the process of self-discovery, and on deep receptivity without retaliation, manipulation or fear of being either taken over or summarily abandoned. That at least is the aim---though not even therapists are perfect. The ending of this experience marks the start of 167 hours without it, of working at being her own therapist, parent, big brother and elder sister while coping with all the various competing demands of her environment until the next session.

The length of time allotted to the session is one of the predictable boundaries of the work of analytical music therapy. As far as is humanly possibly it should remain the same. The patient has the responsibility of arriving on time and the therapist has the responsibility of telling the patient when it is time to leave. The inexperienced music therapist may worry that he has not rounded off the session harmoniously and so prolong the hour, arousing a feeling of insecurity about predictable boundaries in the patient, and creating havoc in his own working schedule. The therapist must try and judge whether the patient is able to contain and work with the tensions thrown up by a session. In this connection, if the patient is out of hospital it is worth enquiring whether she has, or encouraging her to have, some sort of regular routine in her life. It is much easier to cope with the possibly ensuing storms of emotional experience when there are normal everyday things to be done which create a reaassuring rhythm to life.

The therapist can only realistically offer one hour's work in the time allotted, he cannot resolve all dissonances and provide a perfect cadence to every session. Nor indeed should he, for this would lead to the patient permanently opting out of the responsibility of managing herself and her life and projecting this caring, containing part of her personality permanently on to the therapist---a regressive step which would not help the progress of the treatment.

I have found that a full hour is necessary for this work. I used to work three hours at a stretch taking one patient after another but I do not recommend this. One needs a break of about fifteen minutes, or ideally half an hour, in between sessions to write up notes and attend to one's own bodily needs. In my book, Music Therapy in Action (Priestley, 1975), I described how in my early days as an analytical music therapist, I treated a patient who persuaded me to take her on a taximeter system. She would have as long as she felt she needed, provided I did not have other engagements, and pay by the begun half hour. Her longest cathartic session, mostly of crying, was three and a half hours. It may have done something important for her, I can't be sure, but on the other hand I feel that she may also have been deprived of the opportunity to develop her own powers of holding. I would not do that today.

If the patient reaches the end of the session in a regressed, emotional state, it is, of course, necessary to take a few minutes to call to the adult self. It helps to clarify what has been happening, for example by saying, "You have been experiencing the wild jubilations of your four year old self but now it is time to reclaim your adult self and go home, so we will take a few minutes to help you to do this." The therapist has to think where the patient is going and how she is going to get there. Obviously less care needs to be taken with a hospital patient who is just going back to the ward, though an explanatory phone call to the Sister might not be out of place. The private patient, who may have to make a long journey home by car or public transport, needs to be in command of her adult self when leaving. Although one may have left one's own analytic therapy more than once with tears streaming down one's cheeks, I think the pre-verbal quality of music therapy demands that we need to take a little extra care of our patients. In a severe case of one patient close to a psychotic area, I even skipped the music and took her out of the work room and gave her a cup of tea, speaking of everday things until she regained her composure for the hour and a quarter's journey home.

Occasionally a patient will not leave at the end of a session. In this case the therapist can sit down with her for a minute or two getting behind her feeling of how difficult it is to leave and possibly later explore how much she would like to be the therapist's child or companion and stay there permanently. When they feel that their feelings are understood rather then rebuffed in a rational way, most patients will get up and go without further protestations, though I recently heard a Jungian analyst say that she once had to call the police to remove a private patient who refused to leave the premises.

Usually, after a week or two, patients come to the session bursting with things that they want to talk about but sometimes they get to this stage after a difficult silent beginning. However, it is not usually wise to delay the improvisation for more than half an hour or twenty-five minutes because the discussion following the improvisation can be particularly fruitful, often following a completely different direction.

Some patients repeatedly keep the more emotive material until the end of the session. I had one hysterical patient who spent the whole session working up a verbal crescendo until she got to the point one minute before the end of the session, and we had no time for music. I took this up with her and there was some improvement so that we had time for our improvisations once more. But finally, one day she said as she was leaving, with her coat on, that she had no more money for treatment. I offered her two free sessions in which to discuss her feelings about earning money and arranging for a larger allowance from her husband and she accepted this. These were two fruitful and interesting sessions when it emerged that she considered that only work done for love was worth having, and she had successfully manipulated me into giving her this. I told her to go away and see how she got on and whether she felt she needed further treatment. If she could organise a reliable source of payment we could discuss the matter again.

In some cases, such as with a full-time student or a patient on social security, I have agreed to continue treatment for a token payment. But this patient did not work, lived in a nice house with a garden and had one teenage child. Her husband, who was separated from her, was a professional man with a good job. She was making a bid for being taken on as a child which I felt was unhealthy to encourage.

Some patients are adept at finding methods of prolonging their sessions. One woman of forty-five, who was intermittently suicidal with rapid moodswings, used to pour all her depressive material out during the session then, when she was putting on her coat, she would tell me all the encouraging things she had done which I was seduced into taking time to listen to. Again I had to take this up with her in the next session. It sometimes takes the therapist a little time to see what is going on between him and the patient, until a mounting crescendo of irritation tells him that he must clarify the situation for himself and then speak about it. This time it turned out that she felt so guilty at having this time just for herself, that she felt that she had only to present the depressive side of her life; and so she was giving me a very one-sided view of her situation without this prolongation. Now, many years later I found myself shouting at my holistic therapist "Do you think I pay you all this money to tell you how happy I am?" But of course it is most unhealthy for both therapist and patient for the latter not to give a balanced view of her situation.

Some patients prolong the session by getting lost in the music. They will not stop playing. In this situation I glance at my watch and calculate the length of time necessary to discuss the music then first of all make musical gestures at ending the music, something in the nature of a Beethoven symphonic ending. If this fails I stop. If they still continue---and often they do---then I say "We'll have to leave it there so we have time to discuss our experience," or something like that. Please understand that these are guidelines and I still don't get it right all the time. Sometimes there is no time for music because one is concentrating on the music in the words, sometimes no time for ensuing discussion, sometimes no money and sometimes no patient.

It is amazing how, at the end of a session, the patient seems to be able to talk without ever stopping to draw breath to give you a chance to say "Time!" This is only a problem for the hypersensitive therapist but if he reinforces it with an action such as going to stand by the door the patient will usually understand that this is a firm boundary. On re-reading this I discovered that the reason I did not actually do it myself was that the cupboards in my work room are so arranged that if I stand by my door no one can get out.

Yet another complication is with patients who pay at the end of every session. Some therapists prefer this method as it avoids the bother of making out bills, and for the impecunious patient it does not seem as if the therapy is as expensive as if they had to part with a whole month's fees at once. Prolonging the session by payment on completion affords great scope to the time-greedy patient. The obvious method is not to have written out the cheque and to take time in asking the date, not having a pen, finding there are no cheques left and so on. Another method is paying cash and asking for change. If the therapist never gives any, but books the surplus towards the next session it usually discourages this. Then there is the time gained by patients who are supposed to pay at the end of their session and don't. Newly qualified music therapists often feel hesitant to remind their patients to pay. I have ready the words: "I wonder why you forgot to pay me today." The reason is not always negative as one might imagine--- feeling that the therapist is too incompetent to warrant payment or gave too poor a session to be rewarded. It may well be the opposite: that the patient would like the relationship to be a friendly one where no money changes hands. The reason for nonpayment can be brought up and discussed in the next session and this seldom fails to remedy the situation after, at the most, two sessions. The obvious answer would seem to be to ask to be paid at the beginning of the session and certainly if there is lengthy business about holiday dates and changing times this is much more sensible. However, this can sometimes give the wrong atmosphere at the beginning of the work. Your own sensitivity and intuition are the best guides.

Another disturbance of the prescribed hour-long session is caused by patients who leave in the middle of the hour. I have found that, apart from the odd agitated depressed person or chronic schizophrenic, this seldom happens in hospital where patients are conditioned to abide by the rules of their very structured day. The very few patients who have left before the end of a session in my private practice have been people who have themselves been anxious about being abandoned, and wanted to communicate this to me by passing to me the feeling of being abandoned. Occasionally a patient will want to rush out in a highly emotional state. A boy in his teens wanted to do this, but knowing that he had a long journey home alone, I persuaded him to stay and play some pentatonic music which calmed him down, and then we were able to speak about the cause of his distress. However, it is amazing how emotional some patients can be in their session and yet be able to find the adult self who can easily cope successfully with their journey home. The therapist will have to assess carefully each patient's strengths and weaknesses in this connection and this is another reason for hearing the good news as well as the problems.

Suicidal attempts can be another occasional attack on treatment. As soon after the attempt as the patient is able, the therapist can use the music to bring out her murderous rage. Often such patients are cut off from all their feelings, in which case the therapist can say that they have been pushed into him and play this in music. This is, in fact, the truth, for it is no joke to be burdened with this kind of fury after a patient's suicidal attempt. In between weekly sessions it is sometimes necessary and helpful to give the suicidal patient a specific time to ring back to get some forward-moving direction into her thinking. I personally have never had a patient who misused the knowledge of my private phone number in this way although with a certain type of insatiable person I can see that this might happen; and a colleague of mine working with psychopathic people had to have her phone number made ex-directory for this reason. Well, yes, one client did ring at three in the morning when I happened to be going to the bathroom. When I answered it he sounded most disappointed saying that he just wanted to talk to my answering machine.

In cases of acute suicidal crisis, I have found it useful to talk to the patient on the phone for a short while and then give her a physically rewarding task such as having a cup of coffee or having a bath and then letting her ring again. This brings a moment of normality into the patient's life and a moment of physical well-being. It is the nearest thing to being able to care for her in a maternal way. I learnt the hard way to keep at home the addresses of all hospital out-patients to whom I had given my phone number when I was trying to get the home address out of a fading overdosed patient who phoned me at home one evening. In this case I actually misheard the name of the road, but having told her to drink eight glasses of warm salt water, leave the front door open amd give her small son paper and chalks, experienced ambulance men managed to reach and revive her anyway. You may well say that this is hardly analytical music therapy but it does lift one's morale to have one's patient alive for the next session.

Patients may have other reasons for, and other methods of, breaking off treatment. In private practice there is the reason of not being able to afford it. As with the patient described previously, the therapist can allow a small number of free, if necessary, sessions in which to discuss the facts and feelings about the earning, priorities in spending and management of money. Sometimes if a patient is working well in the treatment and has a genuine need, the therapist may feel able to carry one or two such cases without charge, possibly temporarily. Freud initially set aside a couple of hours a week for such cases but found that it changed the therapeutic relationship to such a degree that he no longer found it useful.

Sometimes a patient develops paranoid feelings about the treatment. She believes that the therapist is somehow pushing painful feelings into her, whereas she herself has become strong enough to allow these repressed or suppressed emotions to surface but is projecting them on to her therapist. Where there is a good working alliance the therapist, with a firm holding approach, can discuss this with a patient. Without a good working alliance the patient may just leave suddenly, convinced that the therapist is bent on driving her mad.

With a few patients, the beginning of the work proves so threatening to them that all their symptoms cease and they take what psychoanalysts call a "flight into health." A patient of mine, who had survived analytical music therapy for three years, was referred to the therapeutic community of the hospital where I worked. She survived there for only two and a half days and then absconded and flew to her former home overseas.

With most patients a moment will come when both therapist and patient feel that the patient is ready to continue her journey alone. It is most satisfactory if the patient voices this first. Often it accompanies a new milestone in life, such as a marriage, a new home or job or the passing of an examination---any kind of coming of age.

However, some patients do not feel that they ever want to leave. They want to remain permanently attached to the therapist in the manner of a child or spouse. In this case, when the therapist feels that the separation will be helpful, he can ask the patient to choose a date some way ahead towards which they will work constructively.

Sometimes a patient seems to have gone as far as she can for the moment and the therapist may give reasonable notice of a separation. After a year or six months she may ask to come back and will often use the sessions much more profitably. In three cases where this happened to me, the patients had developed considerably in the interim period and worked much more seriously after the break.

Something should be said about the therapist's absences, too. The therapist would do well to avoid taking on new patients within six to eight weeks of his holiday, particularly the long summer break. But if this is unavoidable it should be discussed thoroughly beforehand in a preliminary assessment session. Treatment is sometimes unavoidably broken by the therapist's illness. There is often, on the part of the patients, a great deal of anger at abandonment, and guilt because aggressive phantasies towards the therapist, as parent in the transference, seem to have come true. These feelings should not be glossed over though the therapist can acknowledge that these patients may also have felt, or shown, genuine concern for his well-being. Brief temporary absences of the therapist, such as missing a week to attend a conference, going to the door or answering the phone and so on, can usefully be discussed, as they often bring up keen irritation; and these feelings can be worked through helpfully before the more serious unavoidable separations and absences of life occur.

Every ending is also a beginning, and if the ending of a session or a treatment enables a fruitful beginning to be made, then it is a successful step in the progress of life.

The following poem was a gift to me from a client who was approaching the end of her six and a half year treatment. Besides being a sensitive and lovely poem, it is an interesting natural example of the therapist's function becoming internalised and the management of loss by introjection. Of course it takes scant account of her negative feelings for me along the way, which we both realised were there and were violently expressed on the cymbal, but then it is the function of art to conceal as well as reveal.

BIRTHDAY GIFT

Housed in my heart
Are hidden melodies,
Unspoken thoughts--
Buried treasure
Over which,
Miser-like
I crouch and gloat.

"Mine alone"
Triumphantly I've said
On many a day,
Caressing my blue and silver jewels:

"No-one knows but me,"
I've whispered,
As my cheeks burned with shame,
Gazing at some tarnished bauble.
"Not worth giving"
I have thought
Glancing at the useless,
Dry and withered piece of love
Lying forlorn and unused in the darkest,
Deepest depths of my being.

This then is my secret core,
My closed book--
Unopened by any,
Yielded to none--
BUT
You came into my life--
Unwanted.
You made me feel pain--
Unforeseen.
You taught me that people
Are human--and precious.

You continue to affirm me
As a loving--and lovable person.

You have opened my eyes
To the joy of sharing--
And the pain and sorrows
Of loneliness
You have created for me
Beautiful silences,
Downy-lined, like a bird's nest.

You have supported me
In hours of darkness,
Strengthened me
In moments of weakness,
Encouraged me to live
When I wanted to die,
Tended my wounds
And lanced my boils.
Shown no revulsion
At my shameful deeds.

You have accepted me
As I am,
Tried always to understand
And given me courage
On this dark voyage
Of self-discovery.

Now, as the time nears
For us to part,
When I may never
See you again,
In my innermost heart,
My secret, inviolable sanctuary,
Seated at ease there,
I find you.

Essay Thirty-One

Postlude: The Ineffable

This is the end of the book---the final essay. I thought I had said enough but, after hearing what he described as a beautiful improvisation on Separation by myself and a flautist from Berlin, Dr. Redfearn asked me why I had never described the beauty of the music and the marvelous mingling of the voices. I answered that it was not usual for performing musicians to speak of such matters. After a sublime rendering of some master quartet, they are to be found discussing their mortgages or playing a game of cards. Ascending to the heights necessitates good earthing. Some things cannot be spoken about, I said. They are not exactly secret, but to immobilise them in words would be not only to destroy them but also to destroy something vital in the performer. I was actually quite frightened of writing this postlude.

Where music flows words cannot follow; to pull music down to the level of words would take the power from it. Music is composed of a multi-dimensional movement of changing pitch, of changing harmony, of subtle alterations of rhythm, of variations in tone colour---and behind this is the inaudible music which carries it all along: the movement of the hearts of the performers. (I am speaking metaphorically here, I do not want any psychologists coming along to ask if they can measure such movements with mechanical instruments, though I feel sure that such movement exists somewhere, possibly clothed in other concepts). How can one take a verbal "still" of the heights of musical relationship in any way that will reproduce its humbling, elevating, brooding, roaring, melting, mysteriously peaceful and explosively joyful qualities? I do not know, nevertheless I agreed reluctantly to try and write this essay.

Not all improvisations have the quality Dr. Redfearn described. About eighty-five percent are quite humdrum affairs, often however, accompanying quite important insights. Some of them are also, musically speaking, quite abysmal. The patient gives the therapist nothing to build on or get hold of and the therapist may stumble from one miserable musical cliche to another desperately searching for a thread to guide him. This is the music of the desert places, and it too has its place in the exploratory journey.   It means something to traverse them together.

A colleague of mine asked how music can be mundane and humdrum. Some of it is. Such music does not penetrate the depths or rise to the heights, nevertheless it can operate as a valuable matrix for holding the emotions, thus enabling images and memories to come forth. Some music is even a kind of anti-music. With patients it can act as a plug to prevent live music from welling up in their inner selves.   A defence against music can be just as effective as when rationalisation prevents the emergence of insights about unconscious impulses. With composed music it can be an inane background which prevents one reaching down to the depths or up to the heights.   And many people use it for just this purpose: to block out the more challenging emotions and keep their minds on a reassuringly humdrum level. Maintaining the humdrum helps to carry out the mundane tasks which take up a great deal of the average person's free time and are so difficult to carry out when one sinks into queer states of mind which involve the outer levels of emotion or the solution of imponderable questions such as four year old children pose before breakfast: "How do you know you are you?" and "Who made God?" and so on.

This kind of defensive music is the very opposite of the kind that I am going to endeavour to describe. I hope the reader will forgive my stumbling efforts to express experiences for which, to my way of thinking, words seem totally inadequate. Be patient, we are approaching the ineffable.

Sometimes, when the therapist and patient are improvising there comes a moment when the music starts to change its quality so that it begins to hold the therapeutic couple. The therapist may feel that the music has become greater than the two of them and then he feels that it is playing him. In fact, instead of being the player he feels that he has become the instrument. At such a time there may be an alteration of consciousness with the act of playing the music with his fingers on the piano creating the lower end of a quivering continuum, reaching up to a lofty area of feeling and thought in quite a different climate. The two players are strangely united in, but overshadowed by, the music. One comes out of such an experience altered, one has lost some of one's constricting individuality and gained a feeling of a greater breadth of being. Usually, not much is spoken after such an improvisation but there is often a look which passes between the two as if to say "We know, we have been there" with often a little half smile and sometimes a sigh of repletion. But is this feeling really shared? I will consider this later.

If one reflects on the two sorts of time, the passing time in which we hurry along to our next pay day and the Eternal Now where we stand still and wonder, I would say that this "receptive creative experience" (RCE) takes place in the Eternal Now. Thus, in a long day of therapy, such moments, though intense, are truly refreshing being deeply rich in meaning. Music, at such times, creates us, we no longer create it.

This RCE is not a state that can be consciously willed, although there must be a certain empathy and openness to experience in the two players. But no expectations or fixed ideas can produce this strange fusion and turning inside out of the creativity. It happens when it happens and if we reach out to meet it there is deep and marvelous magic. We cannot congratulate ourselves, we cannot claim it as our own accomplishment. It is like finding ripe wild raspberries in a strange wood---a rare gift. What can one say? We were there, it came to meet us, we reached out our hands and something happened. For a moment---(or was it a year or a thousand days?), we were transformed. Our doing was done to us.

This kind of music seems to be experienced in an extra dimension. The awareness of body movements and the ensuing sound is the same in all kinds of improvisation but with RCE there can be a sense of the environment closing in with heightened tension (of course you get this in some fine concerts) or a reaching up into a psychic area of light and freedom into which the sounds leap with ecstatic excitement and the two players become not one but three, again the third being the containing matrix of the music's wholeness. It is as if the music were already composed and with each note one is guessing correctly what must follow. The exhilaration is enormous and there is a sense that one has not failed in some great task. (I will not say "succeeded" for the success seems too precarious for that). These moments are naturally sacramental. I do not know what the inward and spiritual grace is but it is a very real presence.

Some people may think of RCE in terms of what Jung described about the joining of animus and anima and giving birth to the Heavenly Child. In the Psychology of the Transference, Jung (1946) quotes from the Rosarium, "In the hour of the conjunction the greatest marvels appear," adding, "For this is the moment when the filius philosophorum or lapis is begotten." And RCE has a similar feeling about it.

But I prefer to think that it is some kind of enchantment. Sometimes the therapist is acting on the patient with sweet and sad sounds, but during the RCE they form a unit of dual enchantment, and yet each is ravished, not by the other but by the greatness of the third aspect which suddenly contains the two. Perhaps I had better come down to earth with actual physical sensations. It is rather like trying to describe a sneeze or an orgasm. You can talk about feeling this or that as a prelude, but the actual event is indescribable although it leaves you in no doubt about whether or not you had it.

Without quoting any of these particular attempts to describe the RCE, I asked two colleagues if they had had such experiences with patients. In reply, one of them said, "Oh, you mean when the music seems to be playing you, oh yes." He knew at once what I was talking about. The other one said she had not had such experiences with patients (it is notable that she specialises in taking very damaged patients) but she felt this in concerts and while practising. I doubted whether the practice experience was the same thing but cannot see why I should deny her this personal truth. She spoke of the well-known pianist John Lill talking of going to meet this by holding back and letting the composer speak. One can understand this better with composed music but in improvisation there is no already existing music, we are making it up as we go along until that moment when the music flows backwards, the RCE, and plays us.

It is not just in one-to-one therapy that RCE occurs. I vividly remember a small group with a colleague and four or five fairly unsophisticated semi-chronic patients who were in the Assessment Unit of the Rehabilitation Department of the hospital where I work. I was playing the violin while the others played untuned percussion instruments. We started off in a jumbly, disintegrated sort of way and suddenly I found myself playing in a strange tone high up on the A string. There was that feeling of incredible intensity as if we were being closely encircled by a ring of silent listeners and watchers, and then it happened: the group and I seemed to form one instrument and this music played on us. The group followed my smallest gradation of tune or tempo of the violin and something seemed to be pouring this icy, piteous music from my violin to which the group appeared to be listening most intently.

Did we talk about it? Not a word. Although it seemed fairly obvious that we must all have been aware of something for us to play with such unity but perhaps we each felt we had had an odd, rather private, valuable experience and that we had better keep it to ourselves. And so we did. Indeed I have never questioned patients about whether they shared these experiences, words seemed too flat-footed and insensitive as vehicles for these emotions. The music had said it. What more did we need? If questioned, each one would clothe his RCE in his own words. If you can imagine the RCE as a central point and our verbal experiences radiating from it you will see that the verbal descriptions could be miles apart, quite unintelligible to one another and possibly very worrying to the others. I have occasionally had an RCE with a multi-disciplinary group. Again it was never discussed. When you touch the magic you respect its priceless fragility. But the silence was rich.

That description was of the intense, quiet variety of RCE. But I have experienced another kind with certain patients and that is a more Dionysian elated rising of rapturous feeling expressed in notes that play in between or high above theirs. In this there is none of the intense feeling of being listened to but a tremendous surge of rising joy and a sense of being in an upper area of delight and ease doing a kind of psychic dance to and with the music. There is a moment of choice before the leap. It takes courage. But once taken it will be sought again when the moment seems ripe. Sometimes, too, when the therapist and patient are improvising, it is as if hordes of dancers are with them or faces seen in the flickering light of the fire. Sometimes in listening to the playback, the client (seldom a patient) will actually dance as the one visible dancer in this invisible throng. Sometimes aeons seem to roll back and we are wandering through strange times and places to collect forgotten treasures of joy and sadness hidden like amber in the sea. Sometimes we seem to be the only performers in some huge awesome place of worship. But usually we are just us in the here-and-now with the music making its subtle alchemical exchange and the patient exclaiming after the playback (as one articulate client did) "But I didn't hear you responding to me while we played. It makes me very happy to hear that."

It can be asked whether RCE contributes anything to the health of the patient. I think it is a by-product of the improvisation, in no way essential for good therapy to take place. Indeed I worked with analytical music therapy for many years before I experienced it. However, it seems to offer the patient on the one hand an experience of tolerable closeness, which he may badly need, and on the other one of tolerable joy, which he also may have lacked. It forms an extension of the normal tuning process which is a function of analytical music therapy, both the individual tuning of the therapist and patient and their tuning one to the other so that emotions may be responded to and resonated, where desirable.

The experiences I have described are quite different from the more chronic countertransference expression which a therapist will play to round out the emotional picture. This always feels to me as if it wells up from below towards the solar plexus and swells like a breaking wave into sound. With this there is none of the strange unity of RCE although the patient will often consciously note what the therapist is doing and resonate to this music which represents his lost or suppressed emotion.

What is certain is that RCE is never experienced in the verbal part of the session. Neither can it be known through reading about it. Some of my readers, however, will recognise RCE as an old and trusted friend for not only can music flow backwards to play the player, but I am assured that art can reach back to create the artist (in fact Picasso said as much), the dance can dance the dancer and poetry can create "living poems" of the poet, so these people may thank me for opening a door to the sharing of such experiences. Others will surely find this whole postlude irritating, woolly and paradoxical. For their sake, I will go no further beyond saying that though these words may be inadequate, with George Lillo I affirm that

> "There's no passion in the human soul,
> But finds its food in music."

References

Alexander, F. & French, T. (1946). Psychoanalytic Therapy (Second Edition). Omaha: University of Nebraska Press.

Alvin, J. (1966). Music Therapy (Fourth Edition). London: John Baker.

Assagioli, R. (1965). Psychosynthesis: A Collection of Basic Writings. New York: Vikings Press.

Barker, C. (1972). Healing in Depth. London: Hodder & Stoughton.

Bartram, P. (1991). Aspects of the Theory and Practice of Music Therapy. Paper presented at the November conference of the Scottish Music Therapy Council, Edinburgh Scotland.

Ben-Tovim, A. & Boyd, D. (1985). The Right Instrument for Your Child: A Practical Guide for Parents. London: Gollancz Press.

Bettelheim, B. (1967). The Empty Fortress. Glencoe: The Free Press.

Bruscia, K. (Ed.). (1991). Case Studies in Music Therapy. Phoenixville: Barcelona Publishers.

Bruscia, K. (1987). Improvisational Models of Music Therapy. Springfield, IL: Charles C.Thomas.

Bion, W. R. (1955). Language and the Schizophrenic. In M. Klein, P. Heimann, and R. Money-Kyrle (Eds.), New Directions in Psychoanalysis, p. 220-239. London: Tavistock Publications.

Bion, W. R. (1959). Experience in Groups. London: Tavistock Publications.

Bion, W. R. (1977). Seven Servants. New York: Jason Aronson.

Brown, D. & Pedder, J. (1961). Introduction to Psychotherapy. London: Tavistock Publications.

Buber, M. (Ed.) (1947). Ten Rungs, Hasidic Sayings. New York: Schoken Books.

Charny, I. W. (1969). Marital Love and Hate. Family Process, 8 (1).

Dicks, A. V. (1983). Marital Tensions (4th edition). London: Routledge and Kegan Paul Ltd.

Frankl, V. (1963). Man's Search for Meaning. London: Hodder & Stoughton.

Feder, S., Karmel, R. L. & Pollock, G. (Eds.). (1990). Psychoanalytic Explorations in Music. Madison, CT: International Universities Press, Inc.

Freud, A. (1936). The Ego and the Mechanisms of Defence. London: Hogarth Press.

Freud, S. (1959). In J. Strachey (Ed.), The Standard Edition of the Complete Psychological Works of Sigmund Freud. London: Hogarth Press & Institute of Psychoanalysis.

Gaston, E.T. (1968). Music in Therapy. New York: McMillan.

Gramlich, E. (1968). Recognition and Management of Grief in Elderly Patients. Geriatrics, 23-87.

Greenson, R. (1967). The Technique and Practice of Psychoanalysis. London: Hogarth Press.

Gris, H., & Dick, W. (1979). The New Soviet Psychic Discoveries. London: Souvenir Press.

Heal, M. (1989). In Tune with the Mind: How Music Therapy Allows the Expression of Inner Feelings. Surbiton: Good Impressions Ltd.

Heal, M. & O'Hara, J. (1993). Therapy of an Anorectic Mentally Handicapped Adult. British Journal of Medical Psychology, 66 (March).

Heimann, P. (1950). On Countertransference. International Journal of Psychoanalysis, 31, 81-84.

Hartmann, H. (1958). Ego Psychology and the Problem of Adaptation (D. Rappaport, Trans.). San Francisco: International Universities Press Inc.

Hoskyns, S. (1988). Studying Group Music Therapy with Adult Offenders: Research in progress. Psychology of Music, 16, 25-41.

Jung, C. G. (1946). The Psychology of the Transference. In H. Read, M. Fordham, & G. Adler (Eds.), The Collected Works of C. G. Jung, 16, 164-323. London: Routledge, & Kegan Paul.

Jung, C. G. (1958). In H. Read, M. Fordham, & G. Adler (Eds.), C.G. Jung: The Collected Works. London: Routledge & Kegan Paul.

Jung, C. G. (1963). Memories, Dreams and Reflections. London: Routledge & Kegan Paul.

Jung, C. G. (1966). The Practice of Psychotherapy. In H. Read, M. Fordham, & G. Adler (Eds.), The Collected Works of C.G. Jung, 16, 353-539. London: Routledge & Kegan Paul.

Khan, H. I. (1960). The Mysticism of Sound. The Sufi Message of Hazrat Inayat Khan. London: Barrie & Rockcliff.

Klein, M. (1931). A Contribution to the Theory of Intellectual Inhibition. Journal of Psychoanalysis, 12, 206-218.

Klein, M. (1955). New Directions in Psychoanalysis. London: H. Karnac Books Ltd.

Klein, M. (1975). Envy and Gratitude. London: Hogarth Press.

Lehtonen, K. (1989). Relationship between Music and Psychotherapy. Paper published by the Faculty of Education, University of Turku, Finland. (A-38).

Lowen, A. (1965). Love and Orgasm. New York: Collier McMillan.

Malan, D. H. (1979). Individual Psychotherapy and the Science of Psychodynamics. Sevenoaks: Butterworth.

Mark, P. (1986). Inner London Probation Service D.T.C., Probation Journal, 33 (December 4).

Mattinson, J. & Sinclair, I. (1979). Mate and Stalemate. Oxford: Blackwell.

Neumann, E. (1973). The Child: Structure and Dynamics of the Nascent Personality (R. Manheim, Trans.). New York: C. G. Jung Foundation for Analytical Psychology.

Odell, H. (1988). A Music Therapy Approach in Mental Health. Psychology of Music, 16, 52-61.

Nordoff, P. & Robbins, C. (1977). Creative Music Therapy. New York: John Day.

Peck, M. S. (1983). The Road Less Travelled. New York: Touchstone Books.

Powell, A. (1983). The Music of the Group: A Musical Enquiry into Group Analysis. Group Analysis, 16, 3-19.

Priestley, J. B. (1964). Man and Time. London: Aldus Books.

Priestley, M. (1975). Music Therapy in Action. St.Louis: MMB Music Inc.

Priestley, M. (1976). Music, Freud and the Port of Entry. Nursing Times, 72 (49), 1940-1941.

Priestley, M. (1977). Music, Freud and Recidivism. Journal of British Music Therapy, 8 (3), 10-14.

Priestley, M. (1978). Countertransference in Analytical Music Therapy. Journal of British Music Therapy, 9 (3), 2-5.

Priestley, M. (1980a). Analytische Musiktherapie und Musikalischer Respons. Musiktherapische Umschau, 1 (1), 21-36.

Priestley, M. (1980b). Analytical Music Therapy and the "Detour Through Phantasy." British Journal of Projective Psychology, 25 (1), 11-14.

Priestley, M. (1983). Analytische Musiktherapie (Brigitte Stein, Trans.). Stuttgart: Klett-Cotta.

Priestley, M. (1985a). Ubertrangung und Genubertragung in der Musiktherapie. Musiktherapische Umschau, 6 (1), 17-36.

Priestley, M. (1985b). Musiktherapie in der Privaten Praxis. Musiktherapische Umschau, 6 (4), 287-296.

Priestley, M. (1985c). Music Therapy and Love. Journal of British Music Therapy, 16 (3), 2-7.

Priestley, M. (1986). Musiktherapie und Liebe. Musiktherapie Umschau, 7 (1), 1-7.

Priestley, M. (1987). Music and the Shadow. Music Therapy: Journal of the American Association for Music Therapy, 6 (2), 20-27.

Priestley, M. (1988a). Music and the Listeners. <u>Journal of British Music Therapy</u>, <u>2</u> (2), 9-13.

Priestley, M. (1988b). Music and the Cycle of Life. Paper presented at the annual conference of the British Society for Music Therapy, November 12, 1988.

Racker, H. (1968). Transference and Countertransference. London: Hogarth Press.

Redfearn, J. W. T. (1992). <u>The Exploding Self</u>. Chicago: Chiron Publications.

Redfearn, J. W. T. (1985). <u>My Self, My Many Selves</u>. London: Academic Press Inc.

Ritchie, F. (1991). Behind Closed Doors: A Case Study. <u>Journal of British Music Therapy</u>, <u>15</u> (2).

Ritchie, F. (1992). Opening Doors: The Effects of Music Therapy with People who have Severe Learning Difficulties and Display Challenging Behaviors. In M. Heal and T. Wigram (Eds.), <u>Music Therapy in Health and Education</u>, 91-102. London: Jessica Kingsley.

Robarts, J. Z. (1992). The Individuation Process Facilitated in Music Therapy with Emotionally and Behaviourally Disturbed Children. Paper presented at the European Community Conference on Music Therapy in Health and Education, Cambridge, England.

Rogers,C. (1965). <u>Client-Centred Therapy</u>. London: Constable Press.

Rogers, P. (1992). Issues in Working with Sexually Abused Clients in Music Therapy. <u>Journal of British Music Therapy</u>, <u>6</u> (2).

Rosenfeld, H. (1955). Notes on the Psychoanalysis of the Superego Conflict in an Acute Schizophrenic Patient. In M. Klein (Ed), <u>New Directions in Psychoanalysis</u>. London: H. Karnac (Books) Ltd.

Rycroft, C. (1972). A Critical Dictionary of Psychoanalysis (2nd edition). London: Penguin Books)

Searles, D. F. (1965). Collected Papers on Schizophrenia and Related Subjects. London: Hogarth Press.

Segal, H. (1964). Introduction to the Work of Melanie Klein (2nd edition). London: H. Karnac (Books) Ltd..

Segal, H. (1979). Klein. London: Fontana.

Scheiby, B. (in press). Death and Rebirth Experiences in Music and Music Therapy. In C. Kenny (Ed.), Listening, Playing, and Creating: Essays on the Power of Sound. Albany NY: State University of New York Press.

Scheiby, B. (1992). Musical Transference and Countertransference: Fellow Travellers or Stowaways on the Musical Journey. Proceedings of the Twentieth Annual Conference of the American Association for Music Therapy: Body, Mind and Spirit: AAMT Coming of Age. Valley Forge, PA: AAMT.

Skynner, A. (1969). A Group-analytic Approach to Conjoint Family Therapy. Journal of Child Psychology and Psychiatry, 10 (October 2), 81-100.

Skynner, A. (1976). One Flesh - Separate Persons. London: Constable Press.

Steele, P. (1984). Aspects of Resistance in Music Therapy: Theory and Technique. Music Therapy: Journal of American Association of Music Therapy, 4 (1) 66-72.

Steele, P. (1988). Children's Use of Music Therapy. Paper presented at the annual conference of the British Society for Music Therapy conference, November 12, 1988.

Steele, P. & Leese, K. (1988). The Music Therapy Interactions of One Session with a Physically Disabled Boy. Journal of British Music Therapy, 1 (1).

Storr, A. (1964). Sexual Deviation. London: Penguin Books.

Storr, A. (1976). The Dynamics of Creation. London: Secker and Warburg.

Storr, A. (1979). The Art of Psychotherapy. London: Heinemann.

Storr, A. (1992). Music and the Mind. London: HarperCollins.

Tao Te Ching (1954). Translated by J. Duyvendak. London: John Murray.

Towse, E., & Flower, C. (1993). Levels of Interaction in Group Improvisation. In M. Heal and T. Wigram (Eds), Music Therapy in Health and Education. London: Jessica Kingsley Publications.

Towse, E. (1991). Relationships in Music Therapy: Do Music Therapy Relationships Discourage the Emergence of the Transference? British Journal of Psychotherapy, 7 (4) 323- 330.

Waelder, R. (1939). Psychological Aspects of War and Peace. New York: Columbia University Press.

Walrond-Skinner, S. (Ed.). (1979). Family and Marital Psychotherapy. London: Routledge and Kegan Paul.

Wigram, T., Saperston, B. & West, R. (Eds). (in press). Music and the Healing Process. Chichester: Carden Publications.

Winnicott, D. (1951). Hate in the Countertransference. International Journal of Psychoanalysis, 30, 69-75.

Winnicott, D. (1971). Playing and Reality. London: Tavistock Publications.

Winnicott, D. (1965). The Maturational Processes and the Facilitating Environment. London: Hogarth Press.

Winnicott, D. (1975). Through Pediatrics to Psychoanalysis. In Collected Papers of Winnicott. London: Hogarth Press.

Woodcock, J. (1987). Towards a Group Analytic Music Therapy. Journal of British Music Therapy, 1, 16-21.

Woodcock, J. (1990). Communications through Music: What is Communicated? Paper presented at the annual conference of the British Society for Music Therapy Conference, London.

Wooster, E. G. (1983). Resistance in Groups as Developmental Difficulty in Triangulation. Group Analysis, 16, 30-40.

Wooster, E. G. (1986). Psychotherapy. Student Health Journal of the Association for Psychoanalytic Psychotherapy in the National Health Service,2,2. (London: Psychoanalytic Psychotherapy)

Zinkin, L. (1983). Discussion of Wooster's Paper. Group Analysis, 16, 40-41.